MCQs AND EMIs
for
MRCPsych PAPER 3
Second Edition

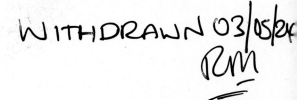

WITHDRAWN 03/05/2

RM

MCQs AND EMIs
for
MRCPsych PAPER 3
Second Edition

Dr. Salman A. Mushtaq
MBBS, MRCPsych, PGDip Derm
Coventry and Warwickshire Partnership Trust

Dr. Imran Mushtaq
MBBS, MRCPCH, MRCPsych, DCH,
PG Dip Child Health, PG Dip-CAMH
Milton Keynes Primary Care Trust

Dr. Imran S Malik
Bsc., MBBS, MRCPsych
Central & North West London Foundation NHS Trust

INTELLECTUAL SIGNATURE SERIES©

First Edition: February 2008 / ISBN-978-0-9558450-0-0
Second edition: August 2008 / ISBN-978-0-9558450-1-7

Notice

The information contained in this book was obtained by the authors from reliable sources. All effort has been made to ensure that the information provided is accurate. However medical knowledge is ever changing and especially in the field of psychiatry there are always some issues where different academics hold different opinions and it's difficult to reach a consensus. Readers are strongly advised to use their judgement and refer to standard text books when in doubt, and update their knowledge according to latest legislation and standards of practice.

No responsibility for loss, damage or injury to any person acting or refraining from action as a result of information contained herein can be accepted by the authors or publishers.

For further details. please contact:
info@intellectualsignature.co.uk

Printing & Production:
Kaghadhi Paerahen

Published by:
Intellectual Signature Ltd.
Registered in England and Wales. Reg No: 06489888
11 Adlington Road
Leicester
Le2 4NA
UK
www.intellectualsignature.co.uk

INTELLECTUAL SIGNATURE SERIES ©

Dedication

It seems like yesterday when we held your hand
to cross the street
thank you for the path you have shown us

TO OUR PARENTS

Mrs. & Dr. Malik Mushtaq Hussain
Mrs. & Dr. Khuda Bakhsh Malik

CONTENTS

INTRODUCTION
Second Edition

Less than six months and we have to write the introduction to the second edition. What can we say, but to show our gratitude to the people who made this book a success. The invaluable feedback we have received from the academics and the trainees simply confirmed that the endeavour was a step in the right direction.

Trainees duly appreciated that we were the only authors who dared to write the first edition of this book before the first exam with a commitment to help trainees. Now that the first exam has been held and in the light of the feedback that we received from respectable academics and more importantly from the trainees, we have further edited the book, included new questions and updated the content to meet the requirements of the trainees, according to the new exam format.

To answer a common question 'will there be questions in exam from this book?' we would like to emphasize that the aim of this book is not to list previous exam questions. Having said that there is a good chance that you will find many similar questions in the exam. If you revise well and practice enough questions, you should be able to answer the exam questions.

Your feedback is our strength!
All the best.

Salman A Mushtaq
Imran Mushtaq
Imran Malik
August 2008

INTRODUCTION
First Edition

Dare we say that there are tough times ahead for Psychiatry trainees? Last year has seen drastic changes to the whole medical profession ranging from changes to the recruitment process to the whole postgraduate medical training. While the survivors struggle to come to terms with the uncertainties of the process, yet again they are faced with another challenge, changes in the requirement, syllabus and exam format of the MRCPsych exam. While all trainees face this new challenge, the trainees facing the real dilemma are the ones who are half way through their training, having passed the part one of MRCPsych exam in the old format and having to prepare for the new Paper 3 (equivalent of part 2 written paper of previous MRCPsych).

With some changes in the syllabus and total change of exam format, currently at the time of writing there is not any book available for the trainees to practice MCQs and exam techniques catering to the new exam format of paper 3.

The previous written paper included Essay paper, Critical appraisal paper and MCQs in the form of extended matching items (EMI) and Individual statement questions (ISQ).

This format is now totally changed to a single paper that will last 3 hours and will include 200 MCQS only, in the form of EMI and Best of five.

Two essential components needed to pass any exam are knowledge and technique. There is a lot of literature available for the trainees to master the theoretical knowledge needed for the exam which like all other trainees we have also used to pass our exams and has proved an invaluable source of references to enable us to compile this book. However the exam technique can only be acquired by practising the

MCQs in the exam format. While there is a pool of EMIs available to practice, the Best of five MCQ format is relatively new for the psychiatric trainees in UK and Ireland with little if any resources available.

The aim of this book is to fill that gap and provide the trainees with a comprehensive resource to practice the new format, best of five MCQs for paper 3 of MRCPsych. Although EMIs are included but main emphasis is on best of five MCQs.

This book is not a substitute for a textbook; instead an exam aid and revision guide for individuals who should have the basic knowledge of the subject as would be expected from a trainee at their current level. Having said that great effort has been put into giving major definitions and explanations of the favourite exam topics for revision and to equip those who might lack some of the necessary knowledge needed to pass the exam.

Primarily this book should provide trainees with enough exam format questions to practice, covering all major topics in the syllabus as per Royal College of Psychiatrists guidelines. Additionally the explanations given with the answers cover all the major topics and should provide an invaluable source of revision material for the MRCPsych exam syllabus, making this book one of its kind catering to the new exam format.

While this book is written for trainees preparing for paper 3 of MRCPsych exam, we sincerely believe that psychiatrists and psychiatry trainees at other levels of training as well as other mental health professionals can equally benefit from this book.

Your feedback is most welcome and will be much appreciated, so as to improve the future editions and other books in this series.

Our sincere wishes and good luck to all the trainees.

Salman A Mushtaq
Imran Mushtaq
Imran S Malik
January 2008

PREFACE
First Edition

How one views professional examinations depends crucially upon position and perspective.

To the patient, examinations are there to guarantee professional competence. However, this is in part a forlorn hope. It is to be regretted that psychiatry advances only slowly and sometimes in a two steps forward and one step back fashion. Nevertheless advance it does. I have long forgotten much of what I learned in preparation for what was the first Royal College membership examination well over thirty years ago. And quite right too. The examination should be a hurdle allowing access for the broadly competent to a career of continuing education.

To the senior doctor, they are remembered as one of the necessary tickets of entry to specialist practice, making sure that only the right people get to join the "club". The examinations of their day tend to be given a rosy or perhaps even a romantic glow. Like the elders of the tribe attending and blessing a hallowed ceremony, they watch the progress of the young initiates through the rites of passage. They mumble memories of how it was in their day remembering the camaraderie and forgetting the pain.

To the educationalist, the construction of such examinations is a challenge and their aim is to discover the extent to which the examinee has or has not attained the objectives of training. However, both the educational expert and the dabbler find only modest consensus as to what these objectives should be and more than modest uncertainty about how their attainment might best be measured. They are subject to the temptation to chop and change both the form and the content of the examination.

To the candidates the examinations are all of the above and much more. Like a big fence in the Grand National, the examinations loom large. Like a tennis match, the candidate tries to respond to everything that is served up. Sometimes it seems impossible although a good technique to cope with this thought is to look around at the people who have passed. Only those with spectacularly low self-esteem will be able to sustain the belief that genius is required. Nevertheless, study is a requisite. And help is welcome. But to whom should the candidate turn?

This book is a useful guide to both the form and content of the MRCPsych examination. It is up to date with the slowly advancing canon of psychiatric knowledge and likewise it is up to date with the more rapidly changing structure of the examination. Crucially it has been created by young psychiatrists who have gone through the process sufficiently recently to be able to know what is useful. They can sustain accurate empathy with those who are preparing to address the examination. As the saying goes these guys have been there and done that and have got the tee shirt.

This book will not prevent the prospective candidate from falling for the temptation to spend all day making a revision plan and thus avoid actually revising. It will not stop everything from yesterday's newspapers to the labels on tomato sauce bottles seeming suddenly to be so much more interesting than psychiatry. But once these demons have been vanquished, the book will be an invaluable resource.
I wish something like it had been around in my day.

Professor Bob Palmer
Department of Psychiatry
University of Leicester
February 2008

ACKNOWLEDGEMENTS

We have been fortunate in having the opportunity to have worked with some of the erudite educationalists and clinicians who inspired us and guided us through our professional career. They encouraged and endowed us with knowledge by virtue of which we have been able to conceive this book. To name only few, Professor Bob Palmar, Prof, Kedar N Dweidi, Dr Rob Holmes, Dr Thavasothy, Dr S Binyon, Dr Chris Mace, Dr S Bhaumik, Dr Roni Taylor, Dr John Milton, Dr Jon Arcelus, Dr J Kenney-Herbert, Dr. A O'Neill-Kerr, Dr. B C Timmins, Dr. R Banhatti, Dr. S Sankar, Dr. K Hadi and Dr. H Vlachos to whom we would like to extend our gratitude for their role in our professional development.

We also feel strongly the need to acknowledge the value of our patients who have been the continuous source of our learning.

Last but not least we thank our wives Sehar, Uzma and Ambreen, and children who exercised extraordinary patience while we were busy in pursuing this venture.

Chapter 1

Questions:
Research Methods,
Evidence Based Practice,
Statistics and Critical Appraisal

1. Which of the following statement regarding confounders is not true?

A. A confounder has a triangular relationship with exposure and the outcome
B. Confounder is on the Causal pathway
C. Negative confounder masks an association which is true.
D. Cofounders are naturally occurring
E. Confounders can be measured and controlled for

2. Which of the following does not reduce confounding?

A. Mantzel-Haenszel test
B. Multiple linear regression model
C. Logistic regression model
D. Stratification
E. Blinding

3. Which of the following statements about randomisation is not true?

A. It ensures that all subjects in a study have an equal chance of being allocated to any group in the study
B. It is the only way to avoid selection bias

C.   Stratified randomisation keeps characteristics as similar as possible across study groups

D.   Concealed allocation checks that the randomisation was adhered to at the time of allocation

E.   Randomisation does not influence the distribution of confounders

4.   Which of the following statements about blinding is true?

A.   Blinding is used at a later stage in the research investigation to avoid bias in the measurement of outcomes of treatment being assessed

B.   It does not include hiding information about the treatment

C.   Single blinding involves hiding allocation information from the assessor analysing the final data

D.   Double Blinding involves hiding allocation information from both the investigator and the assessor analysing the final data

E.   Blinding is not crucial in RCTs

5.   In terms of Reliability which of the following statements is not true?

A.   Reliability describes the consistency of test results on repeated measurements over time or by one or more raters

B.   Reliability cannot be quantified as a correlation coefficient.

C.   Intra-rater reliability of a measure is the extent to which that measure is stable within one rater over time

D.   Inter-rater reliability is the level of agreement between assessments made by 2 or more assessors at the same time.

E.   Split half scale reliability of a measure can be defined as the extent to which that measure is stable between 2 halves of a scale

6.   Which one of the following statements about validity is true?

A.   Validity refers to the extent to which a test measures what it is supposed to measure

B.   Criterion validity is a type of content validity

C.   Face validity is a type of concurrent validity

D.   Convergent validity refers to the extent to which the test is able to distinguish between groups it should theoretically be able to distinguish

E.   Construct validity means simply appearing to be valid

7.   Which of following is true for Intention to treat analysis?

A.   All study participants are included in the analysis if they are eligible patients

B.   All compliant study participants are included in the analysis

C.   All study participants are included in the analysis as long as they are alive

D.   All study participants are included in the analysis as part of the groups to which they are randomised

E.   Excluding patients does not lead to bias

8.   In order to evaluate the local services, all the patients from a hospital were interviewed to comment on the quality of service they received during their stay in the hospital. The study design is:

A.   Cross sectional survey

B.   Qualitative study

C.   Pragmatic trial

D.   Epidemiological study

E.   Prevalence study

9.   Commonly used statistical test for parametric data include:

A.   Mean

B.   Median

C.   Interquartile range

D.   Mode
E.   Frequencies

10.   Which of following is not true for Chi Squared test?

A.   Compares 2 or more groups
B.   Compares between the expected values and the actual
        observed values in a 2x2 table
C.   In Chi Squared test actual numbers are used
D.   In Chi Squared test percentages are used
E.   In Chi Squared test proportions are not used

11.   Skewed data:

A.   Is normally distributed
B.   Can be analysed using parametric tests
C.   Cannot be analysed using non parametric tests
D.   Can be transformed into normal like distribution by
        taking powers, reciprocals or logarithms
E.   Cannot be analysed using tests that don't have the
        assumption of normality

12.   A data is said to be discrete:

A.   If the values or observations belonging to it can be sorted
        according to category, for example colour
B.   If the values / observations belonging to it are distinct and
        separate, i.e. they can be counted (1, 2, 3,.....)
C.   If the values / observations belonging to it can be assigned
        a code in the form of a number where the numbers are
        simply labels. You can count but not order or measure For
        example, in data set males could be coded as 0, females as 1
D.   If the values / observations belonging to it can be ranked
        (put in order) or have a rating scale attached. You can
        count and order, but not measure. For example a rating
        scales of 1,2,3,4 and so on
E.   If the values / observations belonging to it may take on
        any value within a finite or infinite interval. You can count,

order and measure data. For example height and weight

13. You are comparing 2 different interventions, SSRIs and CBT for treating depression. You want to know the results in patients who receive SSRI, patients who receive CBT, patients who do not receive any treatment and the results when both treatments are combined. Which of the following study designs would be most appropriate to answer all your questions?

A. Crossover RCT
B. Parallel RCT
C. Factorial RCT
D. N of one trial
E. Explanatory RCT

14. A Non-parametric test:

A. Needs data to be numerical measurements
B. Cannot use ranked data
C. Cannot be two tailed
D. Usually test median instead of mean
E. Cannot be one tailed

15. Following statements about 'forest plots' are true except:

A. The forest plot is a graph of study outcome on the vertical axis and outcome measure on the horizontal axis
B. The area of the each box represents the weight each study is given
C. When the 95% confidence interval crosses the zero effect line, the study outcome is not statistically significant
D. When z statistic is used, the rule of thumb is that a z value of < 2.2 means that the null hypothesis can be rejected
E. The Mantzel Haenszel procedure is used to produce the final result of a forest plot

16. Analysis of variance:

A.   Can remove systematic variation in a set of data.
B.   Cannot compare means.
C.   Is not based on linear model.
D.   Cannot compare set of experimental treatments.
E.   Is carried out on frequency data.

17.   One- way Analysis of variance:

A.   Is a Non parametric test
B.   Is used when treatments have different variances
C.   Is used to analyse skewed data
D.   Removes one source of systematic variation from the data
E.   Removes two source of systematic variation from the data

18.   A Mean square is:

A.   Is average of all the squares
B.   A sum of squares divided by it's degree of freedom
C.   A sum of squares plus its degree of freedom
D.   A sum of squares minus its degree of freedom
E.   Is a corrected sum of all squares

19.   A new medication for depression is being assessed Volunteers are informed about the effects and possible side effects. Response to treatment is assessed by using MADRS.What study design is this?

A.   Parallel RCT
B.   Factorial RCT
C.   Case series
D.   Open label trial
E.   Ecological study

20.   Randomisation ensures that:

A.   There is no observer bias
B.   There is no publication bias
C.   There is no selection bias

D.   All the confounders are eliminated
E.   That the investigators are blinded to allocation

21.   Two groups are matched for age, sex and genetic
         disposition. One is treated with Anti depressants and the
         other with placebo for 6 months and than treatment
         outcomes are statistically analysed. What type of study is
         this?

A.   Randomised controlled trial
B.   Controlled trial
C.   Case control
D.   Cohort
E.   Pragmatic trial

22.   The power of a test (given all the relevant factors remain
         constant)

A.   Is inversely proportional to the sample size
B.   Is inversely proportional to the significance level
C.   Is directly proportional to the variability of the
         observations
D.   Is represented by confidence interval
E.   Is the chance of rejecting the null hypothesis when it is
         false

23.   Which one of the following statements about Regression is
         not true?

A.   Regression measures the extent to which one or more
         explanatory variables predict an outcome variable
B.   Regression is used to examine the nature of linear
         relationship between x and y
C.   The regression equation represents how much y changes
         with change of x
D.   Regression equation can be used to construct a scatter
         diagram
E.   Regression techniques cannot analyse continuous data

24.   Which of the following statement about Multiple
        Linear Regression is not true?

A.   Is used when there is one explanatory variable
B.   Is a model in which the outcome variable is predicted from
        two or more explanatory variables
C.   The explanatory variables may be continuous
D.   The explanatory variables may be categorical
E.   Is used when the dependent variable may be influenced by
        independent variables

25.   Which of the following statement about P value is true?

A.   P<0.05 means that the probability of obtaining a given
        result by chance is less than one in 2
B.   P<0.05 means that the probability of obtaining a given
        result by chance is less than one in 5
C.   P<0.05 means that the probability of obtaining a given
        result by chance is less than one in 10
D.   P<0.05 means that the probability of obtaining a given
        result by chance is less than one in 20
E.   P<0.05 means that the probability of obtaining a given
        result by chance is less than one in 0.05

26.   You want to compare 2 treatments but want to keep the
        number of patients to a minimum. Which study design
        would you choose?

A.   Cluster randomised trial
B.   Parallel randomised trial
C.   Ecological study
D.   Cross over randomised trial
E.   Cohort study

27.   Crossover trials:

A.   Need more subjects as compared to RCT
B.   Can be used to study the treatment of rare diseases

C.   Does not require the patients to be their own controls
D.   Have problems in terms of matching
E.   Are observational studies

28.   Publication bias:

A.   Is seen in RCT
B.   Is common in controlled trials
C.   Is seen in Meta-Analysis
D.   Is same as Search bias
E.   Is also know as Berkson bias

29.   Berkson's bias:

A.   Is also called Hawthorne effect
B.   Is also called hospital patient bias
C.   Is a type of information bias
D.   Is common in RCT
E.   Is common in Systematic reviews

30.   Hawthorne effect:

A.   Is a type of selection bias
B.   Is also called Interviewer bias
C.   Is also called Ascertainment bias
D.   Is also called Attrition bias
E.   Is also called Simple attention bias

31.   What would increase the power of a study?

A.   Small effect size
B.   Comparing active treatment with placebo
C.   Strict inclusion criteria
D.   Large sample size
E.   Smaller number of subjects

32.   Absolute risk can be defined as:

A. Risk of an event in one group minus the risk in the other group

B. The risk of an event in one group divided by the risk in the other group

C. The probability that the observed difference between the treatments is due to chance

D. The ratio of odds of having the disorder in the experimental group relative to the odds in favour of having the disorder in the control group

E. The number of patients required to be treated with the experimental intervention in order to prevent one additional adverse outcome

33. Sensitivity can be defined as:

A. It measure the proportion of people without a disorder correctly classified by a test

B. It measures the proportion of people with a disorder correctly classified by a test

C. It measures the proportion of people with a positive test result who actually have the disorder

D. It measures the proportion of people with a negative test who do not have the disorder

E. A ratio of the probability of a positive test coming from someone with the disorder compared to one without the disorder

34. Likelihood ratio for a negative test can be defined as:

A. It measures the proportion of people with a positive test result who actually have the disorder

B. It measures the proportion of people with a negative test who do not have the disorder

C. It measure the proportion of people without a disorder correctly classified by a test

D. The likelihood of having the disease as opposed to not having that disease having tested negative for it

E. The likelihood of having the disease, having tested

negative for it

35.   Which one of the following statements about Confidence
        Interval (CI) is true?

A.   It gives the precision of a measure
B.   Is less useful than P value
C.   When quoted alongside a difference between 2 groups, a
        CI that includes one is statistically non significant
D.   When quoted alongside a ratio, a CI that includes zero is
        non significant
E.   The wider the CI, the more confidence we can have in the
        results

36.   Type II error:

A.   Occurs when the null hypothesis is accepted when it is in
        fact true
B.   Occurs when the null hypothesis is accepted when it is in
        fact false
C.   Occurs when the null hypothesis is rejected when it is in
        fact false
D.   Occurs when the null hypothesis is rejected when it is in
        fact true
E.   Is sometimes also referred as false positive judgement

37.   Numbers Needed to Treat (NNT) can be calculated by
        using the following formula:

A.   EER/CER
B.   (CER-EER)/CER
C.   CER-EER
D.   1/ARR
E.   (a/b)/(c/d)

38.   Specificity can be calculated by using the following
        formula:

A. $a/(a+c)$
B. $d/(b+d)$
C. $a/(a+b)$
D. $d/(c+d)$
E. Sensitivity/(1 Specificity)

39. Likelihood Ratio for Positive Test can be calculated by using the following formula:

A. (1 Sensitivity)/ Specificity
B. Sensitivity/(1 Specificity)
C. $a/(a+b)$
D. $d/(c+d)$
E. $a/(a+c)$

40. Which of the following study is most time consuming?

A. Case control study
B. Systematic review
C. Randomised Controlled trial
D. Cohort study
E. Prevalence study

41. Which one of the following statement regarding Survival analysis is not true?

A. It studies the time between entry into a study and a subsequent occurrence of an event
B. Originally such analyses were performed to give information on time to death in fatal conditions
C. They can be applied to many outcomes as well as mortality
D. It cannot be applied to data from longitudinal cohort studies
E. In survival analysis, censored observations make it difficult to determine the mean survival times

42. Which one of the following statement regarding Kaplan-Meier survival analysis is not true?

A.   It looks at event rate over the study period rather than just at a specific time point

B.   It is used to determine survival probabilities and proportions of individuals surviving

C.   It enables the estimation of a cumulative survival probability

D.   Survival curve can take into account censored observations

E.   Time is plotted on the y axis

43.   Which one of the following is not a type of Economic Analysis?

A.   Cost Minimisation
B.   Cost Efficacy
C.   Cost Effectiveness
D.   Cost Utility
E.   Cost Benefit

44-53.   A new screening test for depression is being evaluated. To evaluate it's sensitivity and specificity, it is compared with an established gold standard tool. 300 people are included in the study. They receive the screening test as well as the established test. The results are as follows:

		Gold Standard Test		
		Positive	Negative	Total
Screening Test	Positive	55	45	100
	Negative	20	180	200
Totals		75	225	300

44.   What is the sensitivity of the test?

A.   0.55
B.   0.73
C.   0.82
D.   0.89
E.   0.92

45.   What is the specificity of the test?

A.   0.6
B.   0.7
C.   0.8
D.   0.9
E.   0.5

46.   What is the positive predictive value of the test?

A.   0.40
B.   0.55
C.   0.60
D.   0.65
E.   0.70

47.   What is the Negative predictive value of the test?

A.   0.5
B.   0.6
C.   0.7
D.   0.8
E.   0.9

48.   What is the likelihood ratio for a positive test?

A.   2.50
B.   3.10
C.   3.65
D.   4.65
E.   5.50

49.   What is the likelihood ratio for a negative test?

A.   0.22
B.   0.33
C.   0.44
D.   0.55

E.   0.66

50.   What is the pre test probability?

A.   0.25
B.   0.30
C.   0.35
D.   0.40
E.   0.50

51.   What are the pre test odds?

A.   0.15
B.   0.23
C.   0.33
D.   0.44
E.   0.55

52.   What are the post test odds?

A.   1.00
B.   1.20
C.   2.20
D.   3.00
E.   4.00

53.   What is the post test probability?

A.   0.15
B.   0.20
C.   0.35
D.   0.44
E.   0.54

54.   In Analysis of variance (ANOVA)

A.   Three or more groups are compared on a single continuous measure

B.   Less than three groups are compared on a single
        continuous measure
C.   The groups does not have to be independent
D.   The data used can be non normally distributed
E.   Groups can not be compared

55.   The possibility of publication bias can be evaluated in a
        Meta Analysis by using:

A.   Forest plot
B.   Confidence interval
C.   P value
D.   Galbraith plot
E.   Q statistics

56.   The following statements about 'Funnel plots' are true
        except:

A.   They are also called scatter plots
B.   Larger studies tends to lie on the narrow end of the funnel
C.   Smaller studies tends to scatter more widely at the open
        end of the funnel
D.   Asymmetry at the wide end of the funnel suggests the
        absence of publication bias
E.   Funnel plots can evaluate potential sources of
        heterogeneity

57.   Which one of the following is a Non Parametric test?

A.   Paired t test
B.   Unpaired t test
C.   Wilcoxon matched pairs test
D.   Regression
E.   Multiple regression

58.   Categorical data:

A.   Can be measured on a scale

B.   Have numerical value
C.   Have set values
D.   Are also known as numerical data
E.   Are the same as quantitative data

59.   Which one of the following is not a type of sampling bias?

A.   Hawthorne effect
B.   Berkson bias
C.   Diagnostic purity bias
D.   Neyman bias
E.   Membership bias

60.   John had the following scores in his tests, 13, 6,11,9,8,10 and 7. What is the median in this case?

A.   9
B.   10
C.   6
D.   13
E.   7

Chapter 2

Answers:
Research Methods,
Evidence based Practice,
Statistics and Critical Apprisal

1. B   Confounding can be defined as where a relationship between 2 variables is attributable to a third, relating to both but not on the casual pathway. A positive confounder can result in an association between 2 variables that are not associated. A negative confounder can mask an association, which really exists. Confounders occur naturally and are not created by mistake by researches unlike bias. Confounders must be identified so they can be measured and controlled for. Confounders can be controlled by using several methods like.

1)   Restriction (Inclusion and Exclusion criteria)
2)   Matching
3)   Randomisation
4)   Statistical techniques (multiple linear regression)

> Freedman D 2005, statistical models: Theory and practice. Cambridge University Press

2. E

3. E   Randomisation ensures that all subjects in a study have an equal chance of being allocated to any group in the study thus equally distributing the confounders and avoiding the selection bias. The 3 main types are Simple, Block and

Stratified randomisation. Concealed allocation is used to check that the randomisation was adhered to at the time of allocation. Randomisation is used in RCTs.

Critical Appraisal for Psychiatry by Stephen M Lawrie

4. A   Blinding is used at a later stage in the research investigation to avoid bias in the measurement of outcomes of treatment being assessed. Blinding means that the Patient, investigator and/or assessor do not know what trial treatments are being administered. Blinding can be single where either the investigator or the patient is blind to the allocation, can be double where both the investigator and the patient are blind to allocation or can be triple where the assessor analysing the data is also blind to allocation. There is an overlap with concealment of allocation and blinding though it should be noted that Concealed allocation is different from blinding.

5. B   Reliability can be quantified as a correlation coefficient (Kappa (Cohen's) statistic). Rest of the above statements can be used to define reliability and it's types.

Critical Appraisal for Psychiatry by Stephen M Lawrie, Sackett et al 1991, pp 28-31

6. A   Statement A is the definition of validity. Main types of validity include.

1   Face validity Simply appearing to be true.
2   Content validity The extent to which the test measures variables that are related to that which should be measured by the test.
3   Construct validity - The extent to which the test measures a theoretical concept by a specific measuring device or procedure.
4   Incremental validity - The extent to which the test provides a significant improvement in addition to the use of other approach.

5   Criterion validity. It demonstrates the accuracy of a measure or procedure by comparing it with another measure or procedure that has been demonstrated to be valid. Criterion validity is made up of Predictive validity, Concurrent, Convergent and Discriminant Validity.

7. D   In an intention to treat analysis all study participants are included in the analysis as part of the groups to which they are randomised, regardless of whether they completed the study or not. Excluding patients' leads to bias and intention to treat analysis aims to minimise exclusions and hence bias. The groups that generally tends to be excluded are non compliers, drop outs, ineligible patients and early deaths.

Hollis S and Campbell F, 1999 BMJ, 319:670-74

8. B

9.A   Parametric statistics rely upon assumptions such as independence, equal variance, continuous data and normal distribution.

Wasserman L (2007) All of Non Parametric statistics, Springer

10. C   Chi Squared test is used to compare categorical data from 2 or more groups. In a chi squared test the expected values and the actual observed values are compared in a two by two table. It is carried out on actual number of occurrences and percentages or proportions cannot be used.

Nikulin MS and Greenwood PE (1996) A Guide to Chi Squared testing New York: Wiley Inter science

11. D   Skewed data is defined as asymmetry in the distribution of the sample data values. Values on one side of the distribution tend to be further from the 'middle' than values on the other side. It can be analysed by using non-parametric tests or it can be transformed into normal like distribution by taking powers, reciprocals or logarithms. It

cannot be analysed using parametric tests.

Statistics Glossary v1.1, Valerie J. Easton and John H. McColl

12. B   A is the definition of categorical data. C is the definition of Nominal data. D is the definition of Ordinal data. E is the definition of Continuous data.

Statistics Glossary v1.1, Valerie J. Easton and John H. McColl

13. C   A Factorial design RCT is used when two or more experimental interventions are not only evaluated separately but also in combination and against a control. A 2x2 Factorial design RCT would generate four sets of data to answer the above questions.

14. D   Non-parametric tests can be one tailed or two tailed. They can use ranked data and does not need the data to be numerical measurements.

15. D   z value of > 2.2 mean that the null hypothesis can be rejected.

16. A

17. D

18. B

19. D   In open label trial both the doctors and patients know what treatment is being given. Trial is not blinded. An Open Label Trial can be randomised, or non-randomised, as long as the patients and doctors know what treatment has been assigned.

20. C   Randomisation is a process that ensures that patients in a sample are allocated randomly to different treatments thus preventing selection and allocation bias. It does not prevent observer or publication bias. Randomisation can distribute confounders but not eliminate them.

Investigators are blinded to allocation by blinding and concealed allocation.

21. B

22. E

23. E   Regression analysis is a technique, which examines the relation of a dependent variable (response variable) to specified independent variables (explanatory variables). Regression analysis can be used as a descriptive method of data analysis (such as curve fitting) without relying on any assumptions about underlying processes generating the data. Except E, all the above statements are true

Richard A Berk, Regression Analysis: A Constructive Critique, sage Publication. 2004

24. A   Single Linear Regression is used when there is one explanatory variable. Statements B to E are true. Third type of regression is Logistic regression where the dependent (y) variable is binary.

25. D   P value expresses the probability of getting observed results given a true null hypothesis. P value tells us whether the difference between study groups is due to chance or whether the difference really exists. The results are considered significant if they are unlikely to be due to chance. The P value of less than 0.05 is considered to be significant.

Dallal GE 2007

26. D

27. B   In Cross-over trials all the people receive one form of treatment and than switch to another treatment halfway through the study. The advantages are that they can be used to study the treatment of rare disease, needs less number of subjects than RCT and the patients are their own controls (Perfect matching). Disadvantages are the order effects, carryover effects, historical controls and needs washout period.

28. C   "Publication bias occurs when the publication of research results depends on their nature and direction." It can occur when authors are more likely to submit, or editors accept, positive than negative or inconclusive results. There is a tendency for those negative or inconclusive results to remain hidden and unpublished. Even a small number of such studies can result in a significant bias. This can distort meta-analysis and systematic review of large numbers of studies. Search bias occurs when search is not comprehensive and misses valid studies, which should be included in the systematic review.

BMJ 2005;331:433-434 (20 August), Dickerson K, JAMA 1990; 263(10): 1385-9

29. B   Berkson's bias is also known as hospital patient bias. It may occur when hospital controls are used in case-control studies. If the controls are hospitalised due to an exposure that is also related to the disease under study then the measure of effect maybe weakened, i.e. biased towards the null hypothesis of no association. It's a type of selection bias.

Grimes, A D (2002) Bias and causal associations in observational research. Lancet. Vol 359

30. E   Hawthorne effect is a type of observation bias and is also called 'Simple attention bias'. It usually arises when the subjects change their behaviour due to attention, as they are aware that they are being observed in a study. People generally tend to normalize their behaviour, which can reduce the true association. Ascertainment bias is just another name of Interviewer bias, which arises when the researcher is not blinded to the subject's status in the study and it alters the researcher's approach to the subject.

Attrition bias arises when the number of subjects dropping out of the study differs significantly in the different groups of the study.

31. D   The main factors that increase the power of study or help to achieve adequate power are large sample size, large effect size, high reliability and 0.05 significance level.

32. A

Relative risk: The risk of an event in one group divided by the risk in the other group.

Absolute risk: Risk of an event in one group minus the risk in The other group.

P value: The probability that the observed difference between the treatments is due to chance.

Odds Ratio: The ratio of odds of having the disorder in the experimental group relative to the odds in favour of having the disorder in the control group.

Number needed to treat (NNT): The number of patients required to be treated with the experimental intervention in order to prevent one additional adverse outcome.

Semple D et al (2005)- Oxford handbook of Psychiatry

33. B   (Please refer to answer to question number 34)

34. D

Sensitivity: It measures the proportion of people with a disorder correctly classified by a test.

Specificity: It measures the proportion of people without a disorder correctly classified by a test.

Positive predictive value: It measures the proportion of people with a positive test result who actually have the disorder.

Negative predictive value: It measures the proportion of people with a negative test that does not have the disorder.

Likelihood ratio for a positive test: A ratio of the probability of a positive test coming from someone with the disorder compared to one without the disorder.

Likelihood ratio for a negative test: The likelihood of having the disease as opposed to not having that disease having tested negative for it.

Semple D et al (2005)- Oxford handbook of Psychiatry

35. A The CI can be defined as the range within which the true measure actually lies, with a specific degree of assurance (usually 95%), based upon the estimate from your data set. It gives the precision of a measure. The narrower the CI, the more confidence we can have in the results. CI gives all the information of a P value plus the precision of the estimate. When quoted alongside a difference between 2 groups (e.g. mean, difference), a CI that includes zero is statistically non significant. When quoted alongside a ratio (e.g. relative risk, odds ratio), a CI that includes one is non significant.

Gardner & Altman 1989

36. B Type II error occurs when the null hypothesis (assumption that there is no difference between 2 groups) is accepted when it is in fact false. It is also called false negative. It usually occurs due to small sample size or large variance.

Type I error occurs when the null hypothesis is rejected when it is in fact true, also called false positive. It can arise due to bias or confounding. The probability of making a type I error is equal to the P value.

37. D

Relative Risk (RR) = EER/CER

Absolute Risk Reduction (ARR) = CER-EER

Relative risk reduction (RRR) = (CER-EER)/CER or ARR/CER

Numbers Needed to Treat (NNT) = 1/ARR

Odds Ratio = (a/b)/(c/d)

(CER means control event rate, EER means Experimental event rate. a, b, c and d refer to the values in the corresponding columns in a 2 by 2 table.) Further details about calculating these values can be obtained from several books and websites, for example www.cebm.net

38. B   (Please refer to answer to question 39)

39. B

Sensitivity = a/(a + c)

Specificity = d/(b + d)

Positive Predictive value (PPV) = a/(a + b)

Negative Predictive Value (NPV) = d/(c + d)

Likelihood Ratio for Positive Test = Sensitivity/(1 Specificity)

Likelihood Ratio for Negative Test = (1 Sensitivity)/ Specificity.

Please also refer to answer to question 37.

40. D   Case control and Prevalence studies are relatively quicker to perform. Systematic reviews can take 6 months to 1-2 years and similarly RCTs can take up to few years depending upon the follow up time. Cohort studies are the most time consuming and can be as long as 30 years duration.

41. D   Survival analysis studies the time between entry into a study and a subsequent occurrence of an event. Originally such analyses were performed to give information on time to death in fatal conditions. They can be applied to many outcomes as well as mortality. It is usually applied to data from longitudinal cohort studies. In survival analysis, censored observations and unequal observation periods are potential problems and make it difficult to determine the mean survival times. In such cases the median survival time is calculated.

Jerald F. Lawless. Statistical Models and Methods for Lifetime Data, 2nd edition. John Wiley and Sons, Hoboken. 2003

42. E   The Kaplan-Meier Survival Analysis looks at event rate over the study period rather than just at a specific time point. It is used to determine survival probabilities and proportions of individuals surviving, enabling the estimation of a cumulative survival probability. An important advantage of Kaplan-Meier curve is that the method can take into account 'Censored data. Time is plotted on the x axis and survivors at each time point on the y axis. The Log Rank test is used when Median survival times are compared.

43. B   Economic Analysis is the comparative analysis of alternative courses of action in terms of their costs and consequences.

There are four main types of Economic Analysis:

1)   Cost-minimization analysis. A cost-minimization analysis (CMA) compares alternative programs where all relevant outcome measures are equal (i.e., equal effectiveness or equal patient quality of life). It's the most basic form and simply aims to decide the least costly way of achieving the same outcome

2)   Cost-effectiveness analysis (CEA) compares alternatives and measures (in natural units) the primary objective(s) of the program (i.e., morbidity reduction, life years saved, functional ability on a scale).

3)   Cost-utility analysis (CUA) compares alternatives similar as in a CEA, but uses a more generic outcome measured directly on patients (i.e., quality adjusted life years-QALYs, healthy years equivalent-HYEs). This type of analysis is preferred when there are multiple objectives of a program, when quality of life is an important outcome, and when quality of life and quantity of life are both important outcomes. The primary advantage of a CUA is that the outcome measure is more generic, and this is helpful when comparing the relative merit of many different types of health care programs.

4)   Cost-benefit analysis (CBA), compares alternatives by

using a generic monetary outcome (i.e., £). The indications for using CBA are similar as for CUA (i.e., when there are multiple objectives of a program), the main difference being that the subjective judgements regarding the value of health outcomes are made by techniques like willingness-to-pay (WTP) rather than by utilities (QALYs, HYEs).

44. B

Sensitivity = a/a+c = 55/75 = 0.73

45. C

Specificity = d/b+d = 180/225 = 0.8

46. B

PPV = a/a+b = 55/100 = 0.55

47. E

NPV = d/c+d = 180/200 = 0.9

48. C

LR+ = sensitivity/1- specificity = 0.73/1-0.8 = 0.73/0.2 = 3.65

49. B

LR- = 1- sensitivity/specificity = 1- 0.73/0.8 = 0.27/0.8 = 0.33

50. A

Pre Test Probability = a+c/a+b+c+d = 75/300 = 0.25

51. C

Pre test odds = pre test probability/1- pre test probability

$= 0.25/1 - 0.25 = 0.25/0.75 = 0.33$

52. B

Post tests odds = Pre test odds x LR+ = 0.33 x 3.65 = 1.20

53. E

Post test probability = post test odds/ 1+ post test odds = 1.20/1+1.20 =0.54

54. A ANOVA is a statistical test where three or more groups are compared on a single continuous measure. The groups must be independent and the data normally distributed and at least interval.

Critical Appraisal for Psychiatry by Stephen M Lawrie

55. D Funnel plot and Galbraith plot can be used to evaluate the possibility of publication bias in a meta analysis, though Galbraith plot requires adaptation. Confidence interval measures the estimate of precision. Q statistics is a test for heterogeneity. P value gives you the probability that the observed results of a study can be due to chance. Forest plot is graphical representation of meta-analysis.

56. D Funnel plots are used to evaluate the possibility of publication bias as well as evaluate the potential sources of heterogeneity. In the absence of publication bias the plot resembles a symmetric funnel. Asymmetry at the wide end of funnel is due to absence of small negative results (studies) suggesting the presence of publication bias.

57. C Parametric tests are Mean, standard deviation, Paired t test, Unpaired t test, one way analysis of variance, McNemar's test, Pearson's, Regression and Multiple regression. Non Parametric tests are Median, Interquartile range, Mann Whitney U test; Wilcoxon matched pairs test, Kruskal Wallis analysis of variance, Chi Squared test and

Spearman rank.

58. C   Types of data can be divided into Categorical and Quantitative. Categorical can only have set values of whole numbers. It cannot be measured and has no numerical value. It can be further divided into Nominal and ordinal. Quantitative data is also known as numerical data and can be distributed normally and non-normally. It's subdivided into discrete numerical data and Continuous numerical data.

59. A   Bias can be defined as any process at any stage of inference which tends to produce result or conclusion that differ (systematically) from the truth. Bias can come from number of different sources and should be minimized with on a RCT. Randomisation and Blinding are key mechanisms to reduce bias. Most important type of bias are SELECTION bias, OBSERVATION bias, PERFORMANCE bias, and ATTRITION bias. Selection bias can be further divided into Sampling bias, which is introduced, by the researchers or Response bias, which is, introduced by the study population. Examples of sampling bias include Berkson's bias, Diagnostic purity bias, Neyman bias, Membership bias and Historical control bias. Example of observation bias include Interviewer bias, Recall bias, Response bias and Hawthorne effect.

60. A   Median is the middle number. Important to remember is that first you have to arrange the numbers in ascending order. (6,7,8,9,10,11,13).

·———·

Chapter 3

Questions:
General Adult and
Rehabilitation Psychiatry

1.   A 42 year old man with chronic schizophrenia on
        flupenthixol decanoate depot injection fortnightly had his
        last depot injection 2 days ago from his community
        psychiatric nurse (CPN). At the time CPN did not have
        any concerns regarding his mental state. Today he
        presents to your psychiatry walk in centre where he is
        noted to be confused, disorientated to time and person,
        agitated, continuously drinking water and is repeatedly
        going to toilet to pass water. What is his blood test likely to
        reveal?

A.   Toxic levels of flupenthixol decanoate
B.   Illicit substances
C.   Hyperkalemia
D.   Hyperprolactinaemia
E.   Hyponatraemia

2.   A 34 year old male with hyperthyroidism and residual
        symptoms of schizophrenia had been on maximum dose
        of quetiapine which was changed to risperidone 6 days
        ago, presented with muscle rigidity, hyperthermia, labile
        blood pressure, tachycardia, incontinence, delirium,
        leucocytosis, abnormal LFTs and increased CK. What is
        the likely diagnosis?

A.   Thyroid crisis

B.   Serotonin syndrome
C.   Prolactinoma
D.   Neuroleptic malignant syndrome
E.   Myocardial infarction

3.   Which of the following is not a good prognostic factor in
        schizophrenia?

A.   Living in a developing country
B.   Family history of affective disorder
C.   Marked mood disturbance
D.   Male sex
E.   Higher IQ

4.   A 45 year old African woman who recently moved to UK
        and has been living alone, presents with a 4 month history
        of believing that her neighbour is always looking for an
        opportunity to harm her. She has reported this to police on
        numerous occasions but police was unable to find any
        evidence. Mental state examination is otherwise
        unremarkable. What is the most likely diagnosis?

A.   Paranoid Schizophrenia
B.   Delusional Disorder
C.   Paranoid Personality Disorder
D.   Acute and Transient Psychotic Disorder
E.   Schizotypal Disorder

5.   Which of the following is not a symptom of postpartum
        psychosis?

A.   Mood disturbances
B.   Thoughts of infanticide and/or suicide
C.   Severe cognitive deficits
D.   Occasional hallucinations
E.   Delusions

6.   A 25 year old male presents with low mood, anhedonia,

poor concentration, weight gain, excessive feeling of cold and bradycardia. What is the most likely primary diagnosis?

A. Porphyria
B. Atypical depression
C. Adrenal dysfunction
D. Hypothyroidism
E. Hyperthyroidism

7. A 25 year old Asian lady, victim of domestic violence, presents with symptoms of insomnia, headache, weight loss (BMI 17.5), unable to eat due to nausea, ringing in ears, weakness, tiredness and muscle ache. All investigations regarding physical health are normal. What is the most likely diagnosis?

A. Depression
B. Somatisation disorder
C. Anorexia nervosa
D. Personality disorder
E. Chronic fatigue syndrome

8. Which of the following is true for depression?

A. 30% of patients will have chronic course of illness
B. Risk of relapse is higher in younger patients with the initial acute onset of illness
C. Neuroticism is a poor prognostic factor
D. Suicide rate for severe depressive episode is up to 5%
E. Suicide in severe depressive episode is 10 times more likely than general population

9. Which of the following statement is true with regards to management of depression?

A. Risk of suicide decreases in early stages of antidepressant treatment

B.   Following hospital discharge risk of suicide decreases
C.   Psychotherapy is beneficial in severe depression
D.   Combination of pharmacological and psychological treatment has a synergistic effect in mild to moderate depressive episodes
E.   Combination of pharmacological and psychological treatment in initial stages may complicate the matters and hence should not be used

10.   Electroconvulsive therapy (ECT) is recommended in which of the following conditions?

A.   Maintenance therapy in depressive illness
B.   Prolonged manic episode
C.   Schizophrenia
D.   Recurrent depressive episode
E.   Severe OCD

11.   Which of the following is not a risk factor for completed suicide?

A.   Elderly
B.   Single, divorced or widowed
C.   Female sex
D.   Recent bereavement
E.   Dependence on illicit substances

12.   A 22 year old female with schizoaffective disorder takes risperidone and citalopram. Her citalopram was increased from 40mg to 60mg two days ago. She presents with shivering, fever, diarrhoea, agitation, confusion, hyper-reflexia and ataxia. What is the most likely diagnosis?

A.   Neuroleptic malignant syndrome
B.   Serotonin syndrome
C.   Metabolic syndrome
D.   Malignant hyperthermia

E.   Sepsis

13.   If lithium level is above 4 mmol/L then which of the following is appropriate?

A.   Rehydration
B.   Correction of electrolytes
C.   Dialysis regardless of any clinical symptoms of toxicity
D.   Dialysis only if clinical symptoms of toxicity present
E.   No action required

14.   Which of the following is true for bipolar affective disorder?

A.   Male sex is a good prognostic factor
B.   Within the first 2 years of first manic episode 20 % of patients experience another episode
C.   Depressive features between periods of mania and depression is a poor prognostic sign
D.   30% have regular relapses
E.   Cycling between mania and depression usually decreases with age

15.   With regards to ECT in acute mania which of the following is true?

A.   It is a first line treatment
B.   It has no evidence of any benefit
C.   It should only be used in bipolar depression
D.   It is a treatment of choice in pregnancy
E.   It should not be used in severe cardiac disease

16.   Which of the following patient should be commenced on maintenance treatment for bipolar affective disorder?

A.   First episode of mania
B.   Second episode, first presentation was 10 years ago
C.   Second episode, first presentation was 8 years ago

D.   Second episode, first presentation was 6 years ago
E.   Second episode, first presentation was 4 years ago

17.   After successful treatment with combination of SSRI and
       benzodiazepine when will you consider discontinuing
       treatment in a 21 year old female patient with panic
       disorder?

A.   3 months
B.   6 months
C.   1 year
D.   18 months
E.   2 years

18.   Which of the following is a treatment of choice for specific
       phobias?

A.   Fluoxetine
B.   Benzodiazepine
C.   Propanolol
D.   Behavioural therapy
E.   Psychodynamic therapy

19.   What is the first line treatment for social phobia?

A.   CBT
B.   Behaviour therapy
C.   SSRIs
D.   MAOIs
E.   Beta blockers

20.   Which of the following medical conditions is not
       associated with anxiety like symptoms?

A.   Vestibular nerve disease
B.   Pellagra
C.   Mitral valve disaese
D.   Temporal lobe epilepsy

E.   Hyperparathyroidism

21.   Which of the following is commonly associated with social
          phobia?
A.   Avoidant personality disorder
B.   Schizophrenia
C.   Bipolar affective disorder
D.   Post traumatic stress disorder
E.   None of the above

22.   Which of the following is true for the management of
          obsessive compulsive disorder?

A.   Phenelzine is first line
B.   SSRIs are second line
C.   Clomipramine is third line
D.   Cognitive therapy has proven benefit
E.   Supportive psychotherapy is valuable

23.   Which of the following is not a poor prognostic factor for
          OCD?

A.   Episodic symptoms
B.   Early onset
C.   Longer duration
D.   Bizarre compulsions
E.   Schizotypal personality disorder

24.   A 30 year old female who was involved in a serious road
          traffic accident 10 months ago presents with symptoms of
          insomnia, flashbacks, hypervigilance, exaggerated startle
          response and poor concentration. Which of the following
          will be your treatment of choice?

A.   Fluoxetine
B.   Alprazolam
C.   Trazodone
D.   CBT

E.   Eye movement desensitisation and reprocessing

25.   Which of the following is true for management of anorexia
        nervosa?

A.   Most patients are treated as inpatient
B.   Citalopram may reduce the risk of relapse in individuals
        who had their weight restored in hospital
C.   Individual therapy has no proven benefit
D.   Family therapy is more useful in late onset cases
E.   Serotonin antagonist cyproheptidine may help weight
        gain in restricting type anorexia

26.   Which of the following is not associated with re-feeding in
        anorexia nervosa?

A.   Bloating
B.   Oedema
C.   Dry scaly skin
D.   Congestive cardiac failure
E.   Electrolyte imbalance

27.   Which of the following pharmacological agents does not
        have any beneficial effect in treatment for bulimia
        nervosa?

A.   Fluoxetine
B.   Fluvoxamine
C.   Desipramine
D.   Imipramine
E.   All of the above

28.   Which of the following is the common electrolyte
        disturbance in bulimia?

A.   Hypernatraemia
B.   Hypercalcaemia
C.   Hypokalaemia

D.   Hyperchloraemia
E.   Hypomagnesaemia

29.   Which of the following is the most effective treatment for bulimia nervosa?

A.   CBT
B.   Fluoxetine
C.   CBT combined with fluoxetine
D.   Guided self help
E.   Guided self help combined with fluoxetine

30.   Which of the following is not associated with Kleptomania?

A.   OCD
B.   Depression
C.   Substance misuse
D.   Eating disorders
E.   REM sleep behaviour disorder

31.   A 50 year old female presents with unpleasant, painful sensation in legs particularly at onset of sleep which interferes significantly with her sleep. Which of the following is the most likely diagnosis?

A.   Periodic limb movement disorder
B.   Ekbom's syndrome
C.   Kleine- Levin syndrome
D.   Ondine's curse
E.   Insufficient sleep syndrome

32.   Which of the following should be used in Kleine-Levin syndrome during the periods of attacks of hypersomnia?

A.   Lithium
B.   Carbamazepine
C.   Valproate
D.   Stimulants

E.   SSRIs

33.   Differential diagnosis for REM sleep behaviour disorder
        does not include:

A.   Malingering
B.   Nocturnal epilepsy
C.   Obstructive sleep apnoea
D.   Sleep walking
E.   Insufficient sleep syndrome

34.   Which of the following is a treatment of choice in REM
        sleep behaviour disorder?

A.   Clonazepam
B.   L- dopa
C.   Imipramine
D.   Carbamazepine
E.   Melatonin

35.   Which of the following contributes to a successful
        management plan for personality disorders?

A.   Set goals which are difficult to achieve and then be firm
        with boundaries
B.   Have a short term view
C.   Plan agreed with the patient
D.   Same management plan for all personality disorder
        patients
E.   None of the above

36.   Which of the following is likely cause of rejection for
        treatment of patients with personality disorder?

A.   They are always manipulative
B.   They display disordered attachment in their relationship
        with staff
C.   They are not treatable
D.   There is always a secondary gain involved

E.   All of the above

37.   Which of the following is a main principle of therapeutic community?

A.   Despotism
B.   Bigotry
C.   Communalism
D.   Reality consensus
E.   Blinkeredness

38.   Which of the following is true with regard to psychotherapy in personality disorder?

A.   In DBT patient may contact therapist by phone between sessions
B.   CAT is appropriate for schizotypal personality disorder.
C.   Psychodynamic therapy is of proven benefit in patients with personality disorder
D.   Schema focused CBT disregards early maladaptive schemas and concentrates on new schemas
E.   IPT is contraindicated in patients who have bulimia nervosa with personality disorder

39.   Which of the following should be considered to improve quality of life of a 40 year old male patient with a chronic bipolar affective disorder currently in remission taking lithium 800mg nocte?

A.   Increase lithium dose
B.   Add olanzapine
C.   Interpersonal and social rhythm therapy
D.   Add valproate
E.   Discontinue lithium as currently in remission

40.   What is the main task of recovery in anorexia nervosa?

A.   Restoration of weight

B. Prevent maladaptive behaviours
C. Treating associated OCD
D. Separation of ideas about weight and eating from the wider personal issues and meanings with which they have become entangled
E. Treating associated depression

41. Which of the following is not part of social care needs assessment in chronic mentally ill patients?

A. Patient centred
B. Systematic and repeatable
C. Sensitive to cultural issues
D. Based on patient's deficit
E. Carried out where the patient wishes it to be

42. Which of the following may predict non compliance with medication in a patient?

A. Generalised anxiety disorder
B. Once daily dose
C. Relatively new drug in market
D. Concerns regarding dependency
E. OCD

43. All of the following are principles of evidence-based supported employment except:

A. Vocational rehabilitation is a central component of the work of mental health teams
B. A primary goal of competitive employment in integrated settings
C. Rapid job search with extensive prevocational training
D. Initial and continuing assessment and adjustment
E. Ongoing time-unlimited support and workplace interventions

44. Which of the following is not a role of crisis resolution home team (CRHT)?

A.   Home treatment
B.   Gate keeping
C.   Early discharge
D.   Care coordination
E.   Crisis intervention

45.   A 53 year old, previously highly functional, Caucasian gentleman with no psychiatric history presents with history of progressive ataxia and cognitive decline. He has recently developed urinary incontinence. He has also started believing that his employer and GP are trying to kill him. He does not report anhedonia. He has uncontrolled hypertension and family history of dementia. What is the most likely diagnosis?

A.   Depression
B.   Late onset schizophrenia
C.   Lewy body dementia
D.   Normal pressure hydrocephalus
E.   Vascular dementia

46.   A series of more specific cognitive problems, largely relating to memory and executive function, have now been well replicated as associated with which of the following?

A.   Depression
B.   Bipolar Affective Disorder
C.   Schizophrenia
D.   Organic personality disorder
E.   Substance misuse

47.   Which of the following is used as a screening tool in psychiatry?

A.   Simpson Angus Scale (SAS)
B.   MADRS

C.   SANS
D.   Edinburgh Post Natal Depression Scale (EPDS)

E.   BDI

48.   Which of the following is not a polysomnographic finding in depression?

A.   Prolonged sleep latency
B.   Decreased slow wave sleep
C.   Altered REM / slow wave sleep distribution
D.   Increased muscle movement in sleep
E.   Shortened REM latency

49.   Which one of the following is not a feature of chronic fatigue syndrome?

A.   Disturbed sleep pattern
B.   Feeling tired after rest, relaxation and enjoyment
C.   Duration more than 3 months
D.   Exercise makes person more tired
E.   Muscle aches and pains

50.   What is the relative risk of having Ebstein's anomaly, if mother is on lithium in the first trimester of pregnancy?

A.   1.5
B.   2.5
C.   3.5
D.   4.5
E.   5.5

51.   What is a core feature of borderline personality disorder?

A.   Attempts to avoid abandonment
B.   Impulsivity
C.   Poor self esteem
D.   Empty feeling
E.   Self harm

52.   What is the absolute risk of having Ebstein's anomaly, after first trimester exposure to lithium?

A.   1/10
B.   1/100
C.   1/1000
D.   1/10000
E.   1/100000

53.   What is the incidence of neural tube defects in first trimester valproate exposure?

A.   0.5%
B.   1-2%
C.   4-5%
D.   7-8%
E.   9-10%

54.   A 25 year old man wants to take herbal antidepressant. What herb would you recommend?

A.   Ginkgo biloba
B.   Feverfew
C.   Hypericum Perforatum
D.   Echinacea
E.   Goldenseal

55.   What characterises Generalised Anxiety Disorder?

A.   Depressive episodes
B.   Avoidance to reduce anxiety
C.   Persistent anxiety/apprehension
D.   Autonomic hyperactivity
E.   Motor tension

56.   What characterises phobias?

A.   Avoidance to reduce anxiety
B.   Generalisation of phobia
C.   Displacement
D.   Motor tension
E.   Irrational fear

57.   What rating scale would you use in a woman who is being
        treated for post natal depression with fluoxetine?

A.   MADRS
B.   Edinburgh postnatal depression scale (EPDS)
C.   AIMS
D.   BPRS
E.   SAS

58.   Which of the following has no evidence of treatment in
        PTSD?

A.   EMDR
B.   Hypnotherapy
C.   Trauma focused CBT
D.   Mirtazepine
E.   Amitriptyline

59.   Which of the following is most likely to be seen in anorexia
        nervosa?

A.   High oestrogen
B.   Low cortisol
C.   High white cell count
D.   Low triiodothyronine
E.   Hyperkalaemia

60.   Which of the following is true for babies born to anorexic
        mothers?

A.   Large for dates
B.   Have lower APGAR scores
C.   Are born post-term
D.   Have a larger head circumference
E.   No risk of developmental delay

61.   Which of the following is least commonly associated with
        bulimia?

A.   Oesophageal tears
B.   Dental decay
C.   Peptic ulcer
D.   Parotid gland enlargement
E.   Seizures

62.   Which of the following has the best evidence for its use in pre-menstrual syndrome?

A.   Phenalzine
B.   Reboxetine
C.   Amitryptalline
D.   Fluoxetine
E.   Venlafaxine

63.   Which of the following has the best evidence of use in pre-menstrual dysphoria?

A.   Progesterone
B.   SSRIs
C.   Vitamin B6
D.   Bright light therapy
E.   Oil of evening primrose

64.   Which of the following has gelastic epilepsy, precocious puberty and behavioural problems as its features?

A.   Antiphospholipid Syndrome
B.   Morvan's Syndrome
C.   Stickler Syndrome
D.   Pallister-Hall Syndrome
E.   Hypothalamic Hamartoma

65.   A 35 year old female patient with schizophrenia describes that her husband has been replaced by his 'double' who is identical in appearance but is not the same person. What is this phenomenon called?

A. Capgras syndrome
B. Couvade syndrome
C. Fregoli syndrome
D. Othello syndrome
E. De Clerambault syndrome

Chapter 4

Answers:
General Adult and
Rehabilitation Psychiatry

1. E   This is a classical presentation of rare but potentially fatal
water intoxication in patients with chronic schizophrenia.
Cause for this is unknown. It usually presents with
polydipsia, polyuria and hyponatraemia. In severe cases
confusion, seizures, cerebral and peripheral oedema may
also occur. Other medical causes including SIADH,
diabetes and renal failure should be ruled out. Treatment
is by fluid restriction, may require an admission to a
medical ward depending on the severity of
hyponatraemia. Antipsychotic medication may also need
to be optimised.

Ferrier IN: Water intoxication in patients with psychiatric illness. BMJ
(1985).

2. D   It is potentially a fatal condition. Risk factors include high
potency typical drugs, recent or rapid dose change, and
abrupt withdrawal of anticholinergics, agitation,
dehydration, Parkinson's disease, organic brain disease,
alcoholism, hyperthyroidism, mental retardation and
psychosis. Treatment includes withdrawing antipsychotic, monitoring vitals, rehydration, dantrolene and
bromocriptine, sedation with benzodiazepines and
artificial ventilation if required. It usually requires a
medical ward admission. Consider ECT for treating acute
psychosis. Once physically stable, antipsychotic can be

reintroduced gradually.

Levenson JL. Neuroleptic Malignant Syndrome. AJP (1985).

3. D   Other good prognostic factors are female sex, good premorbid functioning, no family history of schizophrenia, minimal comorbidity, lack of negative symptoms and being married.

Semple D et al (2005) Oxford Handbook of Psychiatry, Oxford.

4. B   It is a delusional disorder because the delusion is non-bizarre and has been present for at least 3 months which is the criteria for ICD-10. Moreover the patient described has some of the risk factors associated with Delusional Disorder namely mean age 40-49 years, social isolation and recent immigration.
Other risk factors include family history, low socioeconomic status, premorbid personality disorder, history of head injury, sensory impairment (deafness) and substance misuse. Good prognostic factors include female sex, age less than 30 years, sudden onset, clear precipitating factors, short duration and higher occupational functioning.
Acute and Transient Psychotic Disorder has a variable presentation but resolves in 3 months (ICD-10).
Schizotypal Disorder shares some features of schizophrenia but not hallucinations or delusions.

5. C   Instead it is mild cognitive deficits. Psychotic symptoms usually occur after symptoms of restlessness, agitation, insomnia, lability of mood and mild cognitive deficits. Course of the illness is similar to a mood disorder. It is a psychiatric emergency as 5% commit suicide and 4% commit infanticide.

6. D   There are number of medical conditions which can produce depression like symptoms.

Endocrine disorders other than hypothyroidism which can produce depression like symptoms are adrenal dysfunction including Addison's disease and rarely hyperthyroidism. Among neurological disorders Parkinson's disease, stroke, epilepsy, tumours, multiple sclerosis, Huntington's disease, head injury and dementias are responsible for this where as certain cancers specifically gastrointestinal carcinomas; pancreatic carcinoma classically presents with depression. In addition infections including hepatitis, syphilis and HIV, and metabolic disorders (hypoglycaemia, porphyria, hypercalcaemia) including vitamin B12 deficiency can also give rise to depression. Anaemia and SLE can also give rise to depressive symptoms.

Schmidt RA: Psychiatry Board Review, second edition (2006).

7. A   Patients with depressive disorder may not present complaining of low mood but may consult their GP for other physical health related complaints. Some of these complaints may include insomnia, fatigue or other somatic complaints. On exploration they may admit to low mood but will attribute this to their primary complaint. In elderly patients presentation of depression could be as confusion, agitation and decline in social functioning without any complaint of a mood disorder. One should also be vigilant of any culture specific issues as Asian women usually present with somatic complaints when depressed.

8. C   Other poor prognostic factors include neurotic depression, old age, residual symptoms, slow onset, personality disorder, substance misuse, physical illness, lack of social support and low self esteem. Risk of relapse is greater when there are residual symptoms after remission. 10-20% patients will have a chronic course with persistent symptoms lasting over 2 yrs. Suicide rate for severe depressive episodes is up to 13% (it is 20 times more likely than general population).

Semple D et al (2005) Oxford Handbook of Psychiatry, Oxford.

9. D   Risk of suicide increases both in the early stages of antidepressant treatment and following a hospital discharge, this is because previously patients may have had psychomotor retardation and poor motivation hence unable to act on their self harm thoughts. With partial recovery they are more able to act on their thoughts. Therefore it is vital that during these periods the patient is adequately monitored. Psychotherapy is not indicated in severe depression as patient is not in a position to make use of it.

10. B   It is indicated in conditions where appropriate pharmacological treatment has proven ineffective and the conditions is thought to be life threatening such as severe depression, catatonia, prolonged or severe mania.
Lithium should be stopped before giving ECT. This is because lithium increases the risk of post-ictal delirium. Other medications which should be discontinued are benzodiazepines and anticonvulsants as they increase seizure threshold.

NICE Guidelines on the use of Electroconvulsive therapy (May 2003).

11. C   Other risk factors for completed suicide include male sex, living alone, low socioeconomic class, unemployed, poor social support, history of suicide attempt, diagnosis of a mental disorder (greatest risk in major depression and anorexia, then functional psychosis, then neurotic and personality disorders), recent inpatient psychiatric treatment and concurrent physical illness.

12. B   It is a rare but potentially fatal syndrome. Its incidence rate is approximately 1 %. It usually requires admission to a medical ward for supportive treatment. Occasionally serotonin receptor antagonists (cyproheptadine, chlorpromazine, mirtazapine, methysergide and propanolol) may be required.

Other than the obvious difference of association with antipsychotics for neuroleptic malignant syndrome (NMS) and an association with selective serotonin re-uptake inhibitors for serotonin syndrome (SS) the other major differences between NMS and SS are that the former has a slow onset and progression with severe muscle rigidity and bradykinesia where as the later has a rapid onset and progression with less severe muscle rigidity and hyperkinesias.

Sorenson S (2002) Serotonin Syndrome. Utox Update, issue 4, volume 4.

13. C   Generally as a first step lithium should be discontinued and patient should be rehydrated. After this patient should be treated symptomatically, if level is above 3 mmol/L and patient is experiencing severe symptoms then dialysis should be done promptly. However for levels above 4 mmol/L dialysis should be done regardless of any symptoms of toxicity.

Schmidt RA: Psychiatry Board Review, second edition (2006).

14. C   Other poor prognostic factors are male sex, evidence of depression, poor employment history, alcohol abuse, psychotic features and treatment non compliance.

Within the first 2 years of first manic episode 40 to 50 % of patients experience another episode. Majority of patients' symptoms are controlled with lithium with 7% no further episode, 45 % with few more episodes where as 40 % have regular relapse. The cycling between mania and depression usually increases with age.

Semple D et al (2005) Oxford Handbook of Psychiatry, Oxford.

15. D   There is strong evidence to support the use of ECT in acute

mania. However in view of recent NICE guidelines its use is only restricted to patients in which pharmacological interventions have failed or they are not appropriate for such interventions like pregnant women or patients with severe cardiac problems. Lithium is the first line treatment for acute mania with response rate of about 80%.

Mukherjee S et al. Electroconvulsive therapy of acute manic episodes: a review of 50 years experience. AJP (1994).
NICE Guidelines on the use of Electroconvulsive therapy (May 2003).

16. E   Any patient with bipolar affective disorder who has had two episodes within 5 years should be commenced on maintenance therapy. Lithium is the first line maintenance therapy where as the anticonvulsants are the second line. Alternative augmentative agents include calcium channel blockers, thyroid hormones and antipsychotics but the evidence for their use is weak.

American Psychiatric Association. Practice guideline for the treatment of patients with bipolar disorder. AJP (1994).

17. C   Beware of withdrawal symptoms which occur in 10 to 20% of patients, 50 to 70% of patients will show re-emergence of symptoms in which case treatment should be continued for another year before a further attempt should be made to discontinue the treatment. Combination of psychological and pharmacological therapy may show synergistic effect. Behavioural therapy has shown high success rate ranging from 60 to 80%.

Ballenger JC et al. Panic attack and agoraphobia. Treatments of psychiatric disorders, 2nd ed. Vol 2. American Psychiatric Pess, Washington DC (1997).

18. D   An example of behavioural therapy is Wolpe's systematic desensitisation with relaxation after graded exposure. Other methods include flooding, modelling and reciprocal inhibition. Medication is usually not used; rarely benzodiazepine may be used to overcome intense fear to allow exposure to the phobic stimulus. Antidepressants are only used if there is a clear diagnosis of depression secondary to the phobia.

Yujuan Choy et al (2007) Treatment of specific phobia in adults. Clinical Psychology Review Volume 27, Issue 3.

19. A   First line treatment is CBT preferably in combination with either SSRI or MAOI. Among pharmacological agents both SSRIs and MAOIs are significantly more effective. Beta blockers and benzodiazepines can also be used.
If not treated it runs a chronic course where as with treatment response rates are up to 90%. Medication should be continued on long term basis as relapse rates are very high without maintenance therapy.

Prasko J et al (2006) Moclobemide and cognitive behavioral therapy in the treatment of social phobia. A six-month controlled study and 24 months follow up. Neuro Endocrinol Lett.

20. E   Other conditions which cause anxiety like symptoms include cardiac failure, IHD, arrhythmias, hypoxia, pulmonary embolism, asthma, COPD, hyperthyroidism, hypoparathyroidism, hypoglycaemia, phaeochromocytoma, anaemia, porphyria, and carcinoid tumour.
Medications which may produce anxiety like symptoms include antihypertensives, bronchodilators, anticholinergics, disulfiram, antiarrythmics, alpha agonists, anticonvulsants, antiparkinsonians, antidepressants, antipsychotics, thyroxine, antibiotics, chemotherapy and NSAIDs. In addition withdrawal from benzodiazepines and any other sedatives.

Semple D et al (2005) Oxford Handbook of Psychiatry, Oxford.

21. A   Other disorders include alcoholism and depression.

Schmidt RA: Psychiatry Board Review, second edition (2006).

22. E   Behavioural therapy is also useful in managing rituals where as thought stopping technique also has its place in ruminations. However cognitive therapy has so far not proven effective.

SSRIs are used as first line, clomipramine is used as either first line or second line where as phenelzine is used as third line and more so in patients with comorbid panic attacks. Buspirone can be used as an augmentative therapy and antipsychotics can be used where there is comorbid, anxiety, psychosis or tics.

Relapse rates are high for stopping medication therefore it should be continued as long term.

ECT can be used in severe cases resistant to pharmacology and behaviour therapy, and suicidal patients. Psychosurgery (cingulotomy) is used as last resort.

23. A   Other poor prognostic factors include comorbid depression, delusional believes, overvalued ideas, giving in to compulsions and symmetry.

Good prognostic factors include episodic symptoms, a precipitating event and good premorbid occupational adjustment.

20 to 40% have chronic worsening symptoms, 40 to 50% show moderate improvement where as 20 to 30% show complete recovery.

Semple D et al (2005) Oxford Handbook of Psychiatry, Oxford.

24. D   Although EMDR has some evidence but remains controversial, NICE guideline supports its use but trauma focused CBT remains first line. With regards to pharmacological treatment there is some evidence for mirtazepine, amitriptyline and phenelzine. Medications are also used to treat any accompanying symptoms of depression, anxiety, psychosis, impulsivity, hyperarousal and sleep problems.

Post-traumatic stress disorder: The management of PTSD in adults and children in primary and secondary care. Nice Guidelines March 2005.

25. E   Cyproheptidine is an appetite stimulant. It does not influence weight gain in patients, other than who suffer from severe restricting type of anorexia.

Family therapy is more useful in early onset cases. Long term individual therapy may facilitate recovery. In addition self help manuals and psychoeducation are also very helpful.   Inpatient treatment is considered for patients who have physical health complications, resistant to outpatient treatment, rapid weight loss, marked change in mental state, develop psychosis or are at high risk of suicide. On rare instances re-feeding may have to be done by detaining under mental health act.

At least one study has shown that fluoxetine may reduce the risk of relapse in individuals who had their weight restored in hospital. It is however not helpful at low weight.

Palmer R: Helping People with Eating Disorders; A clinical guide to assessment and treatment (2003).

26. C   Bloating, oedema and congestive cardiac failure are symptoms of cardiac decompensation. The risk of cardiac decompensation is significant in the first 2 weeks of re-feeding. This is probably because myocardium is not able to cope with the increase metabolic demand of the body. This is prevented by monitoring patient regularly for tachycardia and oedema, monitoring and correcting electrolytes every 3 days in the first week and then every week during the re-feeding. Daily caloric intake should be increased by 200 to 300kcal every 3 to 5 days until sustained weight gain of 1 to 2 pounds per week is established.

Re-feeding oedema is more common in patients who have history of laxative abuse. It is usually self limiting but in severe cases of potassium sparing diuretics have been found useful.

Palmer R: Helping People with Eating Disorders; A clinical guide to assessment and treatment (2003).

27. B   Most but not all antidepressants which have been adequately tested in bulimia nervosa have shown positive effects. Exceptions include fluvoxamine and mianserine.

The antidepressants which are helpful in bulimia nervosa have real but modest efficacy. Fluoxetine, has the most evidence in the treatment of bulimia nervosa. High doses and long term treatment, at least more than a year, is usually required.

Treatment of bulimia nervosa is generally carried out in outpatients, admission to hospital is only indicated if the patient is pregnant (due to increased risk of spontaneous abortion), suicidal, has comorbid physical health problems or has been resistant to outpatient management.

Palmer R: Helping People with Eating Disorders; A clinical guide to assessment and treatment (2003).

28. C   The common electrolyte disturbances in bulimia nervosa are hyponatraemia, hypokalaemia and hypochloraemic alkalosis. This is due to the excessive self induced vomiting in bulimia nervosa.

Schmidt RA: Psychiatry Board Review, second edition (2006).

29. A   In general there is no doubt that psychotherapeutic interventions, particularly CBT is more effective than drug therapy. Studies have also suggested that there is little to be gained from addition of antidepressant drugs to otherwise adequate psychotherapy. However combination of guided self help and drug therapy may be more effective than either of them alone but it is still less effective than CBT.

Schmidt U (1998) Treatment of bulimia nervosa. In: Hoek HW et al (Editors). Neurobiology in the Treatment of Eating Disorders.

30. E   It is associated with OCD, depression, substance misuse and eating disorders. It may also be precipitated by a loss or a major stress.

Kleptomania is an impulsive disorder in which the person is unable to resist impulses to steal. Stealing is not motivated by personal needs or for money. It is common in women with a mean age of 36 years and is treated with SSRIs, CBT and family therapy.

McElroy SL et al (1991) Kleptomania: a report of 20 cases. AJP.

31. B   It is also called restless leg syndrome. An important differential diagnosis is antipsychotic induced akathisia. It is associated with periodic limb movement disorder, uraemia, Parkinson's disease, pregnancy, folate deficiency and iron deficiency anaemia, peripheral neuropathy, poliomyelitis, hypothyroidism and medication related.

It is managed by stimulation of legs by walking, exercise, massage etc. In addition clonazepam can either be used alone or with bromocriptine or opiates.

Periodic limb movement disorder is usually reported by the spouse or partner who shares bed with the individual. It is characterised by repetitive limb movements during night and excessive somnolence during the day. It is common in people over the age of 60 years. It may be associated with use of lithium or tricyclics. Treatment is usually by removing the cause or with clonazepam.

Ondine's curse is also called congenital central hypoventilation syndrome (CCHS) or primary alveolar hypoventilation. A homeobox gene PHOX2B can be associated with CCHS. It is a respiratory disorder which can be fatal if untreated. The sufferer gets a respiratory arrest during sleep because he or she fails to develop autonomic control of breathing. Some patients have down slanting eyes, a small nose, a triangular shape mouth and ears that are low set and rotated backwards.

Todd ES et al (2006) Facial phenotype in children and young adults with

PHOX2B-determined congenital hypoventilation syndrome: quantitative pattern of dysmorphology. Pediatr.Res. 59 (1): 39-45.

32. D   It is a rare syndrome in which a young adolescent goes through episodes of hypersomnia and hyperphagia. Stimulants are only useful during the periods of attacks where as lithium, carbamazepine and valproate are used for prevention only. Frequency of the attacks decreases over years and eventually stop.

33. E   Other differential diagnoses include intoxication, sleep terror and nocturnal dissociative disorder.
         In REM sleep behaviour disorder patient has vivid violent dreams, acts out on dreams whilst asleep resulting in injuries to oneself and the partner sharing bed.

         Schenck & Mahowald.(2002) REM sleep behaviour disorder: clinical, developmental and neuroscience perspectives 16 years after its formal identification in SLEEP. Sleep.

34. A   Clonazepam shows long term and sustained benefits. All the others listed can be used as an alternative to clonazepam. Other measures in managing REM sleep behaviour disorder include treating any primary organic cause and making sure that the sleeping environment is safe for both the patient and the partner.

         Schenck & Mahowald (2002) REM sleep behaviour disorder: clinical, developmental and neuroscience perspectives 16 years after its formal identification in SLEEP. Sleep.

35. C   In addition there should be realistic goals, plans tailored to individual patient's needs with a long term view and a consistent approach to follow the agreed plan across the service.
         Possible treatment goals could include treating axis I disorder, maintaining therapeutic alliance, crisis intervention, understanding difficulties, harm reduction, anger management, developing social skills, addressing substance misuse, motivation enhancement and practical

support.

Davison SE. Principles of managing patients with personality disorder. APT (2002).

36. B They usually generate negative feelings in staff or people who try to help them because of the disruptive and uneasy relationships they develop with them. Therefore it is important to be mindful of this when managing these patients. However this must be made explicit that psychiatric services cannot take responsibility for all adverse behaviours.

Adshead G (1998) Psychiatric staff as attachment figures. Understanding management problems in psychiatric services in the light of attachment theory. BJP.

37. C Other main principles of therapeutic community include democratisation, permissivenessand reality confrontation.
There are a number of modes of interactions between staff and patients in the therapeutic community, namely, various groups and individual sessions during which these principles are achieved. There is evidence that in some patients with personality disorder therapeutic community based management is effective.

Davison & Tyrer. Psychosocial treatment in personality disorder. In personality disorders: diagnosis, management and cause. Ed. Tyrer P. Oxford: Butterworth Heinemann (2000).

38. A Some patients with borderline personality disorder benefit from CAT and DBT. Psychodynamic therapy has no proven benefit in personality disorder however some modified approaches are being used for borderline and narcissistic personality disorders. There is a view that in severe personality disorder psychodynamic psychotherapy should be contraindicated. In schema focused CBT early maladaptive schemas and behaviours are identified and modified.

Davison & Tyrer. Psychosocial treatment in personality disorder. In personality disorders: diagnosis, management and cause. Ed. Tyrer P. Oxford: Butterworth Heinemann (2000).

39. C Maintenance medication should be used at the minimal effective dose where as interpersonal and social rhythm therapy is useful in keeping the mood stable by having a regular daily activity and keeping an optimal level of stimulus. In addition they may also benefit from family therapy, social needs assessment and appropriate community support to keep their life as normal as possible.

40. D In addition tasks of recovery in anorexia include restoration of weight and style of eating that will sustain it and getting life on the move again developing more adaptive ways of dealing with difficult issues in life.

Palmer B. Come the revolution. Revisiting: the management of anorexia nervosa. APT (2006).

41. D Instead it should be based on patient's strengths rather than deficits. In addition it should also be multidisciplinary and reflective, comprehensive, ongoing, and subject to multiprofessional reviews.

Davenport S. Ensuring the community cares: assessment and evaluation of social care needs in long term mental illness. APT (2006).

42. D Other patient factors include young age, complex medication regimen, concerns of side effects, few perceived benefits, stigma of medication and misunderstanding instructions. Severe illness in particular depression, psychosis and cognitive impairment may also predict poor compliance with medication.

Mitchell & Selmes. Why don't patients take their medicine? Reasons and solutions in psychiatry. APT (2007).

43. C Other principles of evidence-based supported employment include rapid job search with minimal prevocational training, and attention to users' preferences and choices.

Studies indicate that using programmes with these characteristics around 58% of people with serious ongoing mental health problems are able to acquire and retain employment.

Crowther et al. Helping people with severe mental illness to obtain work: systematic review. BMJ (2001).
Rinaldi & Perkins. Vocational rehabilitation. Psychiatry (2004).

44. D Care coordination is a role of community mental health teams (CMHTs) where the patient has long term needs and requires close follow up in community, one member of the team is assigned as a care coordinator.

CRHT service is mainly for adults (16 to 65 years old) with severe mental illness; (e.g. schizophrenia, manic depressive disorders and severe depressive disorder) with an acute psychiatric crisis of such severity that, without the involvement of a crisis resolution/home treatment team, hospitalization would be necessary.

The main aims are act as a 'gatekeeper' to mental health services, rapidly assessing individuals with acute mental health problems and referring them to the most appropriate service. For individuals with acute, severe mental health problems for which home treatment would be appropriate, provide immediate multi-disciplinary, community based treatment 24 hours a day, 7 days a week. Ensure that individuals experiencing acute, severe mental health difficulties are treated in the least restrictive environment as close to home as clinically possible and to reduce out of area treatments. If hospitalisation is necessary, be actively involved in discharge planning and provide intensive care at home to enable early discharge.

Early intervention services (EIS) are aimed at people aged

14-35 with first presentation of psychotic symptoms, usually during the first 3 years of psychotic illness. Early treatment is crucial because evidence suggest that the first few years of psychosis carry the highest risk of serious physical, social and legal harm and intervening early in the course of the disease can prevent initial problems and improve long term outcomes. Main aims are to reduce the stigma associated with psychosis and improve professional and lay awareness of the symptoms of psychosis and the need for early assessment. Reduce the length of time young people remain undiagnosed and untreated, DUP (duration of untreated psychosis).

Assertive Outreach Teams (AOTs) are suitable for adults aged between 18 and approximately 65 who have severe and persistent mental disorder (e.g. schizophrenia, major affective disorders) associated with a high level of disability. Usually there is history of high use of inpatient or intensive home based care (for example, more than two admissions or more than 6 months inpatient care in the past two years).One of the criteria involves detention under mental health act on at least one occasion in last 2 years.

Helping people through mental health services' National Audit Office report Dec 2007 www.nao.org.uk.

45. D   In this case the patient has the classical triad of cognitive decline, ataxia and urinary incontinence present in normal pressure hydrocephalus (NPH). Management is usually removing the cause of it which in 50% of cases is a mechanical obstruction in the flow of CSF. In remainder of the cases where NPH is due to idiopathic causes a ventriculo-peritoneal shunt is put in place, this usually results in reversal of the symptoms.

46. C   With regards to cognitive disorders in schizophrenia, several studies have noted problems in attention, declarative memory, and higher-order problem-solving.

These deficits appear at the onset of the illness and are stable throughout. There is also increasing evidence that these deficits are related to abnormalities in the frontal and limbic brain structures, and genetic markers. Atypical antipsychotic medications, cognitive enhancers, and cognitive rehabilitation have shown some benefit.

Hoff et al. Neuropsychology in schizophrenia: an update. Schizophrenia. Current Opinion in Psychiatry. (2003).

47. D The Edinburgh Postnatal Depression Scale (EPDS) has been developed to assist primary care health professionals to detect mothers suffering from postnatal depression. Previous studies have shown that postnatal depression affects at least 10% of women and that many depressed mothers remain untreated. The EPDS consists of ten short statements. The validation study showed that mothers who scored above threshold 92.3% were likely to be suffering from a depressive illness of varying severity. A careful clinical assessment should be carried out to confirm the diagnosis. The scale indicates how the mother has felt during the previous week and in doubtful cases it may be usefully repeated after 2 weeks. The scale will not detect mothers with anxiety neuroses, phobias or personality disorders. The EPDS may be used at 6-8 weeks to screen postnatal women. The child health clinic, postnatal check-up or a home visit may provide suitable opportunities for its completion.

Montgomery-Asberg Depression Rating Scale (MADRS) is a clinician-rated scale. It is designed to be used in patients with major depressive disorder, both to measure the degree of severity of depressive symptoms, and particularly as a sensitive measure of change in symptom severity during the treatment of depression.

Simpson-Angus Scale (SAS) is a clinician-rated scale. It is designed for assessing parkinsonian and related extrapyramidal side effects.

Beck Depression Inventory (BDI) is intended to assess the

severity of depression in diagnosed adults and adolescents 13 years of age and older. It is not meant to serve as an instrument of diagnosis, but rather to identify the presence and severity of symptoms consistent with the criteria of the DSM-IV. It must not be used as a sole diagnostic measure.

SANS assesses a wide variety of different negative symptomatology, specifically in individual group measures. It has been shown to retain validity in a variety of different cultural settings.

48. D Increased muscle movement in sleep is a polysomnographic finding in panic disorder. All the other findings listed in the question are present in depression and to a lesser degree in dysthymic disorder.

Edward C et al. Guide to Neuropsychiatric Therapeutics. Lippincott Williams & Wilkins (2006).

49. C The duration has to be 6 months. Other common names for chronic fatigue syndrome include myalgic encephalomyelitis, post- viral fatigue syndrome and neuromyasthenia. It is a diagnosis of exclusion. It is more common in women between the ages of 40 and 50 years. It presents most commonly with severe mental and physical exhaustion which does not improve with rest. In addition there are other symptoms present which may involve multiple systems including gastrointestinal, endocrine, autonomic, cardiac and respiratory problems, myalgia, low immunity, depression and cognitive dysfunction. There is no real consensus over treatment but commonly used therapies include CBT and graded exercise therapy (GET). Only 5-10% of patients fully recover.

Carruthers BM et al (2003 Myalgic encephalomyelitis/chronic fatigue syndrome: clinical working definition, diagnostic and treatment protocols. Journal of Chronic fatigue Syndrome.

50. C However 95% confidence interval for this is very wide

(0.1-8.4). Because in past the lithium baby register was a voluntary reporting system and only positive cases were reported therefore earlier studies have overestimated the incidence of Ebstein's anomaly. The rate of Ebstein's anomaly in general population is 1:20000 in live births.

Warner, James, P (2000) Evidence Based Psychopharmacology 3. Assessing evidence of harm: What are the teratogenic effects of Lithium Carbonate? Journal of Psychopharmacology 14 (1).

51. B   Some researchers describe impulsivity or affective impulsivity as a main core feature of borderline personality disorder.

Becker DF et al (2002) Diagnostic Efficiency of Borderline Personality Disorder Criteria in Hospitalised Adolescents: Comparison with Hospitalised Adults. Am J Psychiatry.

52. C   Babies who are exposed to lithium in the first trimester have up to 10 fold increased risk of having congenital anomalies notably Ebstein's anomaly. Birth weights are usually higher in children exposed to lithium during pregnancy.

Cohen L. Lithium and Depakote in Bipolar Disorder Patients of Childbearing Age. Family Practice (2000).

53. B   After first trimester carbamazepine exposure incidence rate for neural tube defects is between 0.5-1.0%.
For all antiepileptic drugs together incidence of congenital malformations is increased about two to threefold. There is no reliable data for individual drugs.

Wiek A. Teratogenic syndromes. In: Adverse syndromes and psychiatric drugs: a clinical guide. Haddad P et al (Editors). (2004).

54. C   Hypericum Perforatum (St. John's Wort) is among the most favourite herbal drugs, and is the only herbal alternative to classic synthetic antidepressants in the therapy of mild to moderate depression. Several clinical studies have been conducted to verify the effectiveness of extracts of Hypericum Perforatum.

As a first step in this patient one should enquire his concerns regarding the allopathic medication and if required he should be reassured. It is also important that he is informed about all the options available to him including social support, voluntary organisations and psychological interventions. Once he is aware of all the options and chooses to use herbal remedy then you may suggest St. John's Wort and encourage him to consult an herbal practitioner. He should also be made aware that St. John's Wort interacts with other medications including warfarin, digoxin, theophylline, cyclosporine, SSRIs and triptans.

Ginkgo biloba improves circulation and delays cognitive decline in elderly.

Feverfew is used in migraine.

Echinacea and Goldenseal are cold remedies.

Wurglics et al (2006) Hypericum Perforatum: A 'Modern' Herbal Antidepressant: Pharmacokinetics of Active Ingredients. Clinical Pharmacokinetics, vol 45.

55. C   The essential feature is anxiety, which is generalized and persistent but not restricted to, or even strongly predominating in, any particular environmental circumstances (i.e. it is "free-floating"). As in other anxiety disorders the dominant symptoms are highly variable, but complaints of continuous feelings of nervousness, trembling, muscular tension, sweating, lightheadedness, palpitations, dizziness, and epigastric discomfort are common. Fears that the sufferer or a relative will shortly become ill or have an accident are often expressed, together with a variety of other worries and forebodings. This disorder is more common in women, and often related to chronic environmental stress. Its course is variable but tends to be fluctuating and chronic.

The sufferer must have primary symptoms of anxiety

most days for at least several weeks at a time, and usually for several months. These symptoms should usually involve elements of:

A.   Apprehension (worries about future misfortunes, feeling "on edge", difficulty in concentrating, etc.);

B.   Motor tension (restless fidgeting, tension headaches, trembling, inability to relax); and

C.   Autonomic overactivity (lightheadedness, sweating, tachycardia or tachypnoea, epigastric discomfort, dizziness, dry mouth, etc.).

The ICD-10 Classification of Mental and Behavioural Disorders, World Health Organization, Geneva, 1992.

56. E   A phobia is an irrational fear of specific objects, places or situations, or activities. Although fear itself is to some degree adaptive, the fear in phobias is irrational, excessive and disproportionate to any actual danger.
The irrational fear, however, must be distinguished from a schizophrenic delusion, which involves a fixed false belief. The person with OCD has multiple fears and phobias, not merely an isolated, circumscribed fear.

Andreasen & Black. Introductory Textbook of Psychiatry. (2006).

57. A   Montgomery-Asberg Depression Rating Scale (MADRS) is a clinician-rated scale. It is designed to be used in patients with major depressive disorder, both to measure the degree of severity of depressive symptoms, and particularly as a sensitive measure of change in symptom severity during the treatment of depression.

Benazzi F. Severity gradation of the Montgomery-Asberg Depression Rating Scale (MADRS) in outpatients. J Psychiatry Neurosci. (1999).

58. B

Post-traumatic stress disorder: The management of PTSD in adults and children in primary and secondary care. Nice Guidelines March 2005.

59. D   In addition to low triiodothyronine in anorexia nervosa, there is oestrogen deficiency, high cortisol, leukopenia and hypokalaemia.

Munoz & Argente (2002) Anorexia nervosa in female adolescents: endocrine and bone mineral density disturbances. European Journal of Endocrinology, vol 147.

60. B   The literature to date concerning pregnancy outcome in women with eating disorders is not definitive. Some studies suggest outcomes such as pre-term delivery, small for gestational age, low birth weights, intrauterine growth restriction and low APGAR scores in babies born to mothers with eating disorders. There is also increased risk for these babies to have smaller head circumference and developmental delay.

Neuhalfen & Bunton. What is the prevalence of birth defects in infants born to mothers with eating disorders, compared to infants born to mothers without eating disorders? Proceedings of 3rd Annual GRASP Symposium, Wichita State University (2007).

61. E   Seizures in bulimia are secondary to hypocalcemia which is usually induced by laxative abuse, and hyponatremia induced by water loading in underweight bulimics.

62. D   Selective serotonin reuptake inhibitors are found to be effective in treating premenstrual symptoms, with continuous dosing regimens favoured for effectiveness. No SSRI is better than other.

Shah NR et al (2008) Selective Serotonin Reuptake Inhibitors for Premenstrual Syndrome and Premenstrual Dysphoric Disorder: A Meta-Analysis. Obstetrics & Gynecology.

63. B

Shah NR et al (2008) Selective Serotonin Reuptake Inhibitors for Premenstrual Syndrome and Premenstrual Dysphoric Disorder: A Meta-Analysis. Obstetrics & Gynecology.

64. E Hypothalamic Hamartoma (HH) is a benign brain tumour, a mass of disorganised neuronal or glial tissue on or near the hypothalamus. It varies in size and is generally not detectable on CT scans or MRIs. It commonly presents with gelastic (laughing) epilepsy. Most cases will present in childhood but onset of epilepsy can occur in adulthood. Most common behaviour disorder includes aggressive behaviour also known as hypothalamic rage. You may see them in neuropsychiatry clinics for epilepsy and cognitive decline. Treatment is antiepileptic drugs and in resistant cases neurosurgery.

HH can be associated with Pallister Hall Syndrome, which consists of multiple malformations, including imperforated anus and polydactyly.

Morvan's 'fibrillary chorea' or Morvan's syndrome is characterized by neuromyotonia, pain, hyperhydrosis, weight loss, severe insomnia and hallucinations.

Pearce JMS (2004) A Note on Gelastic Epilepsy. European Neurology. Vol 52.

65. A Capgras syndrome can be seen in a variety of psychiatric illnesses but 60% of cases are associated with schizophrenia. However it remains a rare symptom of schizophrenia. Fregoli syndrome is the opposite of Capgras syndrome as in this the patient believes that the strangers are 'really' familiar people. This is also a rare a symptom of schizophrenia. Couvade syndrome is not delusional in nature. In this the male partner of a pregnant lady starts experiencing pregnancy related symptoms including nausea, vomiting, cravings and abdominal pain but does not believe that he is pregnant. It is a cultural norm in certain cultures. Othello syndrome is a delusional believe that one' partner is unfaithful. This can occur as a part of psychotic illness, single non bizarre delusion or as a result brain damage secondary to injury or illicit substances. The partner who is alleged to be unfaithful is at a high risk of violence. De Clerambault syndrome is a delusion of love in which the person believes that the other person is in love with them and is destined to be together despite the fact they might have had little or no contact at all. This is also a rare symptom of schizophrenia.

.———.

Chapter- 5

Questions:
Liaison Psychiatry

1. A 20 years old young woman admitted to neurology ward for sudden weakness of her right limb. She does not seem overtly concerned with her illness. What is the most likely diagnosis?

A. Hypochondriasis
B. Malingering
C. Conversion disorder
D. Persistent delusional disorder
E. Factitious disorder

2. A young male patient presents with altered level of consciousness, chewing movements and olfactory hallucinations. Diagnosis of Partial complex seizure was made. All of the following are correct except:

A. Automatism
B. Perceptual alteration
C. Derealization
D. Episodes usually last for 3 minutes
E. Flashbacks

3. Contraindications to sex reassignment surgery (SRS) for transsexuals include all of the following except:

A. Anxiety disorder
B. Substance misuse

C.   Major depression
D.   Psychotic illness
E.   Personality disorders

4.   A 42 years old man with trisomy 21 presents with memory
        difficulties and making frequent mistakes. He is getting
        increasingly forgetful. He has learning disability and is
        under the annual review of a cardiologist. What is the most
        likely diagnosis in this case?

A.   Hypothyroidism
B.   Alzheimer's disease
C.   Intracranial tumor
D.   Wilson disease
E.   Multi-infarct dementia

5.   Recognized features of somatoform pain disorder include
        all of the following except:

A.   Substance misuse is commonly associated
B.   Sickle cell crisis is included in differential diagnosis
C.   High comorbidity with major depression
D.   High comorbidity with psychosis
E.   Classified in DSM-IV as pain disorder

6.   The most common cause of delirium in elderly is:

A.   Polypharmacy
B.   Alcohol abuse
C.   Substance misuse
D.   Vitamin B1 deficiency
E.   Infections

7.   A 35 years old male presents with severe headaches,
        papilledema and homonymous hemianopsia. Which part
        of the brain may be associated with these symptoms?

A.   Frontal lobe
B.   Medulla Oblongata
C.   Cerebellum
D.   Parietal lobe
E.   Occipital lobe

8.   All of the following are true regarding Somatization disorder except:

A.   May be associated in 1-4% of general population
B.   Strong association with personality disorder
C.   Also known as Briquet's syndrome
D.   Complications may result from invasive testing
E.   Association with low stigma

9.   All of the following are correct regarding psychiatric symptoms due to medical conditions except:

A.   According to DSM-IV, the psychiatric presentation of a medical illness is classified as a "mental disorder due to a general medical condition"
B.   There may be atypical presentation of a specific psychiatric diagnosis
C.   Neurosyphilis, once a common cause of admission to mental institutions, is still common despite the invention of penicillin
D.   Multiple sclerosis (MS) is related to multifocal lesions in the white matter of the CNS
E.   Patients with Herpes encephalitis commonly present with bizarre, inconsistent behaviour and a waxing and waning mental status

10.   You are asked see a 27 years old man with anxiety, morning sickness and weight gain for past 3 months, in A&E on medical team's request. His wife is 4 months pregnant. All of the following features will make a diagnosis of couvades syndrome likely except:

A.   Husband of pregnant woman may experiences some
         symptoms of pregnancy
B.   Begins in the end of the first trimester
C.   Only known cure is birth of the child
D.   Insomnia
E.   Extremely rare

11. All of the following statements about temporal lobe
         epilepsy are true except:

A.   Paranoia
B.   Hypersexuality
C.   Simple complex seizure
D.   Hypergraphia
E.   Female patient can feel orgasms while suffering from a
         temporal lobe epilepsy episode

12. All are true regarding association of medical conditions
         with psychiatric symptoms except:

A.   Cushing's disease as high as 20-30%
B.   Hypothyroidism as high as 50%
C.   90% of cases with adrenal disorders
D.   Hyperthyroidism as high as 50%
E.   Hypopituitarism as high as 70%

13. A young woman was admitted to a medical ward with
         anxiety and hyperventilation. While you are explaining
         the recognized features of hyperventilation syndrome to
         the medical students present at the time of your
         assessment, which one of the following features you will
         not mention as a recognized feature?

A.   Respiratory alkalosis
B.   Numbness of fingers
C.   Sudden onset of chest pain
D.   Metabolic alkalosis
E.   Carpopedal spasm

14.   Which of the following statements is not correct regarding brain tumors?

A.   Brain tumors are important cause of psychiatric symptoms

B.   Frontal lobe tumors are responsible for approximately 80% of the patients with psychiatric symptoms

C.   Limbic tumors can produce delusions

D.   Patients with non-dominant temporal lesions can present with memory and speech abnormalities

E.   Hypothalamic tumors can cause affective symptoms such as rage, mania and emotional lability

15.   All of the following are true regarding HIV related psychiatric symptoms except:

A.   Patients with AIDS have psychiatric and neurological symptoms from primary CNS lymphoma

B.   HIV can cause a subacute encephalitis and dementing complex

C.   HIV encephalopathy manifests as a non-progressive subcortical dementia

D.   In the early stages, signs of encephalopathy include difficulty concentrating, subtle mood changes, disorientation, withdrawal, or lethargy

E.   Early therapy with Azidothymidine (AZT), is recommended for HIV encephalopathy

16.   All of the following are recognized in parathyroid disorders except:

A.   Hypercalcemia

B.   Delirium with psychosis is a common presentation of patients with severe hypermagnesemia

C.   Hypomagnesemia occurs in association with hyperparathyroidism

D.   In hyperparathyroidism patients can experience delirium, sudden dementia, depression and anxiety

E.   In hypoparathyroidism, patients most commonly experience delirium

17.   All of the following statements about systemic lupus erythematosus (sle) are true except:

A.   Africans and Asians are often more affected than whites.
B.   Prevalence of neuropsychiatric manifestations is upto 75-90%
C.   The presence of severe depression or psychosis is associated with anti-D antibodies in the serum
D.   90% of cases are in women
E.   Treatment is with high-dose steroids

18.   All of the following statements about Multiple sclerosis (MS) are true except:

A.   30-50% has cognitive deficits
B.   Patients experience euphoria same as in hypomania and is characterized by an unusually cheerful mood
C.   Memory loss is the most common cognitive symptoms
D.   Abstract reasoning, planning, and organizational skills are affected
E.   Major depression is very common in individuals with MS

19.   Sodium imbalance may presents with all of the following except:

A.   Myxedema
B.   Intense anxiety
C.   Rapid correction of hypernatremia can lead to central pontine myelinolysis
D.   Depressed mood
E.   Delusions and hallucinations can also occur with hyponatremia

20.   All are true regarding the clinical manifestations of stages of hepatic encephalopathy except:

A. There are 4 stages
B. Disorientation is observed in stage 2
C. Arousal stupor is associated with stage 3
D. Stage IV Coma
E. Impaired cognition in stage 2

21. The differential diagnosis of psychiatric symptoms in patients with chronic renal failure include all of the following except:

A. Hypercalcemia
B. Hyperphosphatemia
C. Hypernatremia/hyponatremia
D. Hyperglycemia
E. Hypoglycemia

22. All of the following are recognized features of Thyroid disorders except:

A. Symptoms of anxiety, confusion, and agitated depression
B. Psychiatric symptoms usually resolve with treatment of the hyperthyroidism
C. Hypomania and frank psychosis
D. When hyperthyroidism develops rapidly, the psychiatric features are usually delirium and psychosis
E. Stress can precipitate Grave's disease

23. A plastic surgeon referred a 21 years old young woman for psychiatric assessment, as she believes that her ears are too large and wants surgical correction. Which one of the following statements about Body dysmorphic disorder (BDD) is not correct?

A. Gender identity disorder is included in differential diagnosis
B. Obsessive and compulsive rituals
C. High co-morbidity
D. Most common symptom is of nose defect

E.   Without treatment, BDD could be a lifelong problem

24.   Which one of the following statements is not true
        regarding Wernick's encephalopathy (WE)?

A.   In industrialized countries 60-70% of the cases of thiamine
        deficiency are associated with alcohol misuse
B.   Failure to diagnose WE and institute adequate parenteral
        therapy results in death in 20% of patients
C.   75% will be left with permanent brain damage involving
        severe short-term memory loss if untreated
D.   The daily thiamine requirement for healthy individuals is
        between 1-2 mg per day
E.   Presents with nystagmus, gaze palsies, ophthalmoplegia

25.   Recognized features of cerebral lupus include all of the
        following except:

A.   Organic brain syndrome
B.   Depression
C.   Depersonalization
D.   Schizophrenia like presentation which can not be
        differentiated with classic schizophrenia
E.   Psychomotor retardation

26.   All of the following are true regarding HIV/AIDS except:

A.   HIV enters the brain, early in the course of infection
B.   Presence of multinucleate giant cells in brain indicate HIV
C.   CD8:CD4 ratio is a proxy marker for disease progression
D.   Non-Hodgkin's lymphoma is common
E.   Insight is well preserved until late in the course of illness

27.   All of the following are true regarding anorexia nervosa
        except:

A.   Morgan Russell scale is used for outcome measure
B.   It is more common in white females

C. EAT-30 can discriminate well between normal and anorexic patients
D. Premature birth is an independent risk factor
E. Association of OCD

28. A 39 years old woman's MRI shows atrophy of caudal nucleus and putamen. There has been progressive deterioration in her memory & facial and limb movements. Most likely cause for her symptoms is:

A. Alzheimer's disease
B. Wilson disease
C. Huntington's disease
D. Creutzfeldt-Jakob disease
E. Hallervorden-Spatz syndrome

29. All of the following is true regarding risk factors of postnatal depression except:

A. Single mother
B. Young age
C. Severe baby blues
D. Poor social support
E. Family history of depression

30. A 52 years old man presents with daytime drowsiness. Which one of the following statement will make it unlikely diagnosis of narcolepsy?

A. Irresistible urges to falls asleep for briefly during the day
B. Stereotyped, repetitive movements of the legs during sleep, accompanied by brief arousal and sleep disruption
C. Cataplexy
D. Sleep paralysis
E. Hypnogogic hallucinations

Chapter 6

Answers:
Liaison Psychiatry

1. C   Conversion Disorder is a condition where patients present with neurological symptoms such as numbness, blindness, paralysis, or fits, but where no neurological explanation can be found. The ICD-10 classifies conversion disorder as dissociative (conversion) disorder, which suggests the symptoms arise through the process of dissociation.

Stone J, Carson A, Sharpe M., 2005, Functional symptoms in neurology: Assessment, Journal of Neurology, Neurosurgery and Psychiatry (Neurology in Practice); 76 (Suppl 1): 2-12.

2. D   Episode usually lasts between 30 seconds and 2 minutes. Complex partial seizures cause impaired consciousness and arise from a single brain region. Impaired consciousness implies decreased responsiveness and awareness of self and surroundings. Complex partial seizures typically arise from the temporal lobe but may arise from any cortical region. Automatisms are quasi-purposeful motor or verbal behaviour that commonly accompany complex partial seizures.

3. A

sample d, et al (2005) transsexualisms -oxford handbook of psychiatry, oxford.

4. B   This man has Down's syndrome and the likely diagnosis is Alzheimer's disease. Several molecular and clinical similarities have been detected in Alzheimer's disease (AD) and Down syndrome (DS). The most remarkable feature is abnormal accumulation of -amyloid in the brains of both individuals affected with AD and aging DS patients followed by dementia. In addition, AD patients exhibit dermatoglyphic patterns similar to those in DS, and late maternal age is a risk factor in both diseases. AD and DS could be related genetically because AD families exhibit a higher rate of DS cases and vice versa. Although numerous discoveries have been made in the elucidation of the etiopathogenic factors in AD and DS, little progress has been achieved in understanding the origin of the common features of the two diseases.

Petronis A (1999) Alzheimer's Disease and Down Syndrome: From Meiosis to Dementia. Experimental Neurology, Volume 158, Number 2, pp. 403-413.

5. D   It is overrepresented in patients with anxiety disorders, substance misuse and personality disorders.

Sample d, et al (2005) somatoform pain disorder-oxford handbook of psychiatry, oxford.

6. A   One of the most frequent causes of delirium in the elderly is overmedication. The causes of delirium fall into four basic categories: metabolic, toxic, structural, and infectious. Delirium occurs most frequently in the elderly and the young, but can occur in anyone at any age. Of persons over 65 who are brought to the hospital for a general medical condition, roughly 10% show signs of delirium at admission. It is suspected that another 10%-15% may develop delirium while in the hospital.

Curyto K J et al (2001) Survival of Hospitalized Elderly Patients with Delirium: A Prospective Study. American Journal of Geriatric Psychiatry 9; 141-147.

7. E   The occipital lobe is involved in the understanding of visual images and the meaning of written words. Occipital

lobe tumours can present with seizures, visual (more common), auditory, olfactory and tactile hallucinations, impairment of vision and disturbance in motor function.

Sang Kun Lee, et al (2005) Occipital Lobe Epilepsy: Clinical Characteristics, Surgical Outcome, and Role of Diagnostic Modalities. Epilepsia, vol 46;5, 688-695.

8. E   Somatization disorder is a chronic condition in which there are numerous physical complaints. These complaints can last for years, and may result in substantial impairment. The physical symptoms are caused by psychological problems, and no underlying physical problem can be identified. Somatization disorder is highly stigmatized, and patients are often dismissed by their physicians as having problems that are "all in their head."

Noyes R, et al., (2006). "Distinguishing between Hypochondriasis and Somatization disorder: a review of the existing literature". Psychother Psychosom 75 (5): 27081.

9. C   Neurosyphilis is now rare.

10. E   Couvade comes from the french word couvee meaning "to hatch". Couvade is a common but poorly understood phenomenon whereby the expectant father experiences apparently physical symptoms during the pregnancy for which there is no recognized physiological basis. Some researchers estimate that anywhere from 11 to 65 percent of expectant fathers experience some symptoms. Generally, Couvade Syndrome begins in the end of the first trimester and increases in severity until the third trimester. The only known cure for couvade is birth of the child. In some extreme cases, fathers can grow a belly similar to a 7 month pregnant woman and gain approximately 25 to 30 pounds ("phantom pregnancy"). Other symptoms include and are not limited to developed cravings, suffered nausea, breast augmentation and insomnia.

11. B   Hyposexuality is a typical symptom rather than hypersexuality.

12. B   Hypothyroidism as high as 20%.

13. D   Metabolic acidosis is a recognised feature. In the US, as many as 10% of patients in a general internal medicine practice are reported to have, Hyperventilation Syndrome(HVS) as their primary diagnosis. Overall up to 6% of the general population may have this condition to a variable degree. The peak age of incidence is from 15-55 years, but cases have been reported in all age groups except infancy. A female preponderance of HVS cases exists; the female-to-male ratio may be as high as 7:1.

Gardner WN. The pathophysiology of hyperventilation disorders. Chest 1996;109:516-34.

14. D   Patients with dominant temporal lesions can present with memory and speech abnormalities.

15. C   HIV encephalopathy manifests as a progressive subcortical dementia with nonspecific CSF abnormalities and cerebral atrophy with ventricular dilation.

16. B   Delirium with psychosis is a common presentation of patients with severe hypomagnesemia.

Cryer P, Slone R, Whyte M (1996) Depression and hypercalcemia. Clinicopathologic Conference. Am J Med.101(1):111-7.

17. C   The presence of severe depression or psychosis is associated with anti-P antibodies in the serum.

Ainiala H, Loukkola J, Peltola J, et al(2001) The prevalence of neuropsychiatric syndromes in systemic lupus erythematosus. Neurology. 57(3):496-500.

18. B   Multiple sclerosis (MS) is a demyelinating disorder characterized by multiple episodes of symptoms of a neuropsychiatric nature related to multifocal lesions in the white matter of the CNS. Prevalence is estimated to be approximately 50 cases per 100,000 people. Behavioral symptoms in MS include personality changes and feelings of euphoria and/or depression. Approximately 25% of patients experience euphoria that is different from hypomania and is characterized by an unusually cheerful mood.

Rosati G (2001). "The prevalence of multiple sclerosis in the world: an update". Neurol. Sci. 22 (2): 11739

19. C   Rapid correction of hyponatremia can lead to central pontine myelinolysis. Hyponatremia occurs in various conditions. This condition is usually observed in postoperative patients and in patients with severe vomiting and diarrhea, syndrome of inappropriate secretion of antidiuretic hormone (SIADH), extensive burns, cirrhosis, or endocrine abnormalities (eg, myxedema, Addison disease). Hypernatremia usually results from inadequate ingestion of water or from the inability of the kidneys to conserve water. The elderly population is particularly sensitive to dehydration, and elderly persons can have acute mental status changes. As with hyponatremia, the rate of correction of hypernatremia is important. Overly rapid correction can lead to cerebral edema.

Early MRI findings of central pontine myelinolysis following 'rapid' correction of hyponatremia (2004). European Radiology, 14:3.

20. E   Impaired cognition is associated with stage 1. There are 4 stages:

Stage I	Apathy, restlessness, impaired cognition, impaired handwriting and reversal of sleep rhythm.
Stage II	Lethargy, drowsiness, disorientation, asterixis, beginning of mood swings and beginning of behavioural disinhibition.
Stage III	Arousable stupor, hyperactive reflexes

and short episodes of psychiatric symptoms.

Stage IV   Coma (responsive only to pain).

Andreoli T, et al. (1993) Cecil Essentials of Medicine. 3rd ed. Philadelphia.

21. B   Hypophosphatemia is associated with psychiatric symptoms in patients with renal failure.

22. D   When hypothyroidism develops rapidly, the psychiatric features are usually delirium and psychosis, which has also been termed myxedema madness.

Fukao A, Takamatsu J, Murakami Y(2003) The relationship of psychological factors to the prognosis of hyperthyroidism in antithyroid drug-treated patients with Graves'' disease. Clin Endocrinol (Oxf).58(5):550-5.

23. D   The percentage of patients concerned with the most common locations, according to one study, is as follows:
- Skin (73%)
- Hair (56%)
- Nose (37%)
- Weight (22%)
- Stomach (22%)
- Breasts/chest/nipples (21%)

Katharine A. Phillips (2007) Suicidality in Body Dysmorphic Disorder Primary Psychiatry.14 (12):58-66.

24. A   In industrialized countries, 90% of thiamine deficiency cases are associated with alcohol misuse, but it may also occur due to other causes of malnutrition. Other causes of thiamine deficiency may be found in patients with carcinoma, chronic gastritis, or continuous vomiting.

Day, E., Bentham, P., Callagham, R. et al. (2004) Thiamine for the WernickeKorsakoff Syndrome in people at risk from alcohol abuse (Cochrane Review). In The Cochrane Library, issue 2. John Wiley & Sons Ltd, Chichester, UK.

25. D   Schizophrenia like presentation are uncommon and are usually distinguished from true schizophrenia by the presence of visual as well as auditory hallucinations and by an associated disturbance of sensorium with disorientation and confusion.

Vinken PJ, et als . Handbook of clinical neurology. Vol-55, Elsevier Science Publishers, Amsterdam.

26. C CD4:CD8 ratio is a proxy marker for disease progression.

Waldrop-Valverde (2005) Influence of depression and HIV serostatus on the neuropsychological performance of injecting drug users. Psych Clin Neurosci:59(4) 372-8.

27. C Eating Attitudes Test (EAT)-26 is a widely used, standardized, and self-reported questionnaire designed to assess pathological eating behaviours, attitudes, and thoughts. It can discriminate well between normal and anorexic patients.

David M. Garner & Paul E Garfinkel (1979) Eating Attitudes Test- Eating Disorder.
David M. Garner, et al., (1982).

28. C Huntington's disease (HD), known historically as Huntington's chorea and chorea maior, is a rare inherited neurological disorder affecting up to approximately 1 per 10,000 people of Western European descent and is even rare for Asian and Africans. The symptoms of Huntington's disease usually develop when people are between 30-50 years old, although they can start much earlier or much later. The symptoms can also differ from person to person, even in the same family.

The early symptoms include:

- Slight, uncontrollable muscular movements
- Stumbling and clumsiness
- Lack of concentration
- Short-term memory lapses
- Depression

- Changes of mood, sometimes including aggressive or antisocial Behaviour.

Bates, Gillian, Peter Harper, and Lesley Jones (2002). Huntington's Disease - Third Edition. Oxford: Oxford University Press.

29. B   Other risk factors are older age, previous history of depression, poor relationship with owns mother, unwanted pregnancy, other significant psychosocial stressors and previous post-partum psychosis.

Sample D, et al (2005) Illnesses related to childbirth -Oxford handbook of Psychiatry, Oxford.

30. B   Nocturnal myoclonus refers to stereotyped, repetitive movements of the legs during sleep, accompanied by brief arousal and sleep disruption. The main characteristic of narcolepsy is excessive daytime sleepiness (EDS), even after adequate night time sleep. Four other "classic" symptoms of narcolepsy, which may not occur in all patients, are cataplexy, sleep paralysis, hypnogogic hallucinations, and automatic behaviour.

.————.

Chapter 7

Questions:
Forensic Psychiatry

1.   Which is the most common sexual offence?

A.   Rape of a female
B.   Unlawful sexual intercourse with a girl under 16 years of age
C.   Gross indecency with a child
D.   Indecent exposure
E.   Incest

2.   HCR-20 is an empirically guided clinical evaluation for:

A.   Risk of self harm
B.   Risk of vulnerability
C.   Risk of escape from a secure establishment
D.   Risk of violence
E.   All of the above

3.   Which of the following may be responsible for failures in mental health services?

A.   Mental health professional giving too much importance to reports from carers and members of public about disturbed behaviour
B.   Ignoring civil liberties of patients who are at risk of suicide or violent behaviour
C.   A tendency to take a cross sectional rather than a long term view of the risk of violence
D.   Sharing information in the best interest of patient
E.   None of the above

4.   There are about 500 homicides per annum in England & Wales. Which of the following statement is true according to National Confidential Inquiry into Homicides & Suicides?

A.   20 homicides were committed by persons with psychosis
B.   40 homicides were committed by persons with psychosis
C.   60 homicides were committed by persons with psychosis
D.   80 homicides were committed by persons with psychosis
E.   100 homicides were committed by persons with psychosis

5.   Relational security is:

A.   The balance between intrusiveness and openness; trust between patients and professionals
B.   Systems and routines for the control and checking of patients
C.   Secure attachments with family
D.   Risk of violence in relationships among patients
E.   Less important than environmental security

6.   Which of the following is not included in Environmental security?

A.   Structure of the building to prevent absconding
B.   Regular maintenance of the building
C.   Most restrictive environment possible
D.   Design of the building to facilitate good observation
E.   Good standard of decoration as a sign of respect to patients detained within

7.   Which of the following is not true with regard to Procedural security in a high secure hospital?

A.   Visits are by prior written arrangement only
B.   Visitors require identification and pat down searches
C.   Letters and telephone calls in and out are monitored
D.   Legal communication is monitored
E.   All financial affairs are monitored

8. Which of the following is not a sign for diminished need for security for a move from Medium to Low secure unit?

A. Accepts treatment and legal obligations
B. Capable of openness and trust with members of MDT
C. Capable of limited exploration of mental state in relation to risk
D. Can use escorted community leaves sometimes
E. Stable for 6 months

9. Black population is significantly overrepresented in criminal justice system and psychiatric services, and have higher rates of detention under the mental health; this is possibly due to:

A. Psychiatrists have little understanding of the black culture
B. Black population has genetic predisposition to schizophrenia
C. When not well black people can be more dangerous
D. Black people inherit criminogenic behaviour
E. Multifaceted reasons and include both individual and institutional factors

10. A heavy smoker 40 year old male patient with Paranoid Schizophrenia in a medium secure unit maintained on clozapine (plasma levels within therapeutic range) for 3 years and is currently symptom free. The medium secure unit goes smoke free in line with the Government policy. How would you change the clozapine dose?

A. No change as the patient is stable on it
B. Increase the dose by 2.5 fold
C. Reduce the dose by 1.5 fold
D. Increase the dose by 1.5 fold
E. Reduce the dose by 2.5 fold

11. Which of the following antipsychotic has substantial amount of data supporting a threshold target concentration associated with a good therapeutic

response in many patients?

A.   Olanzapine
B.   Risperidone
C.   Amisulpride
D.   Clozapine
E.   All of the above

12. Which of the following is true with regard to Norclozapine?

A.   It is pharmacologically active in humans
B.   Trough plasma clozapine + norclozapine concentration of 0.35mg/L is associated with good response in many patients
C.   Its levels are only useful after clozapine tissue distribution has been completed
D.   Its measurement in conjunction with plasma clozapine provides an index of clozapine N-demethylation
E.   It only gives information on acute exposure of clozapine

13. Which of the following is true with regard to Dangerous and Severe Personality Disorder (DSPD)?

A.   Is recognised by ICD-10
B.   Is recognised by DSM-IV
C.   Refers to people who pose a very high risk of self harm
D.   Is a legal term
E.   Only refers to people with personality disorder who have committed a very serious crime

14. What is the peak age of offending?

A.   14-17 yrs
B.   24-27 yrs
C.   34-37 yrs
D.   44-47 yrs
E.   54-57 yrs

15. Which of the following is true for female offenders?

A. 30% of known offenders are female
B. 41% of convicted women are convicted of theft
C. Women are less likely to be put on probation due to them being highly emotional
D. Women form less than 4% of prison population
E. Women commit more violent crimes than men

16. Which of the following is true with regard to homicides and mental disorders?

A. In 50% of female homicides the offender has a psychiatric condition
B. Women predominate among depressive homicides and the most common victim is their child
C. In men the conjunction of depression and homicide tends to occur in young age
D. In 35% of male homicides the offender has a psychiatric condition
E. Depression is not associated with homicides committed by people with unstable personality

17. What is the phenomenon called in which there is a desire to punish the spouse (usually the husband) by killing the children?

A. Homicide complex
B. Teasing complex
C. Modelling complex
D. Victim complex
E. Medea complex

18. In which one of the following a parent or carer, usually the mother, fabricates symptoms or injuries to the child, and then presents the child for treatment?
A. Munchausen syndrome
B. Munchausen syndrome by proxy
C. Malingering

D.   Conversion disorder
E.   Factitious illness

19.   Which one of the following is true for Rape?

A.   Rarely committed as a direct result of a delusional state or
          hallucinations
B.   Perpetrator has no character disorder
C.   Drug abuse is not common in the perpetrators
D.   Alcoholism is rare in the perpetrators
E.   Some perpetrators show evidence of intense heterosexual
          fears

20.   Which one of the following is true for Penile
          Plethysmography (PPG)?

A.   Measures sexual fantasies
B.   Has shown that there is no difference in sexual arousal
          between rapists and controls
C.   A positive PPG result predicts future behaviour
D.   Has no value in assessment of sex offenders
E.   Can be used to monitor treatment progress in sex
          offenders

21.   Which one of the following is true for antilibidinal
          medication in sex offenders?

A.   Its use requires consent of the patient
B.   Cyproterone acetate is an antilibidinal medication and is a
          control drug
C.   Has no effect
D.   It reduces sex drive by loss of erection
E.   Should be used in all sex offenders

22.   Which one of the following is true for offending in
          schizophrenia?

A.   Violence only takes place in the acute phase of the illness
B.   Violence rarely happens by acting on the delusional

believes
C.   Minor offences are more common than serious offences
D.   Strangers are common victims
E.   Victims characteristics have no contribution to violence

23.   Which one of the following is true for offending in affective disorders?

A.   Offending is more common in depression than in mania and hypomania
B.   Offending is more common in affective disorders than in other functional psychosis
C.   Violent offending is common in depression
D.   Shoplifting in middle aged offenders may be associated with depressive illness
E.   A friend is a usual victim in altruistic homicides

24.   Which one of the following is one of the vulnerabilities that may predispose to violence in schizophrenia?

A.   History of employment
B.   Pre morbid success in education
C.   Personality deterioration
D.   Late onset of substance misuse
E.   Belonged to high socioeconomic class before getting unwell

25.   What should be the main focus of DSPD treatment?

A.   Treating the personality disorder using strict boundaries
B.   Management of the offence related risk
C.   Criminogenic needs only
D.   Violent behaviour and attitudes
E.   Non-criminogenic and criminogenic needs

26.   Which one of the following is true for patients with morbid jealousy?

A.   Carry a high risk of violence to their sexual partner

B.   Psychotic cases have poor prognosis
C.   In light of the principles of confidentiality the potential victim is not informed
D.   It is easy to distinguish between normal and morbid jealousy
E.   The risk to the spouse reduces over time even if not treated

27.   Which one of the following is not part of the fitness to plead test?

A.   Understand the charge
B.   Instruct the lawyer
C.   Challenge the jury
D.   Plead to the charge
E.   Understand the law

28.   What does 'mens rea' refer to?

A.   Automatism
B.   Guilty mind
C.   Automatic behaviour
D.   Automatism simpliciter
E.   Insane

29.   Which one of the following is true for prediction of violence?

A.   Personality traits are the strongest predictors
B.   There are specific predictors for offenders with mental illness in comparison to the offenders who are not mentally ill
C.   One out of every three patients detained on the basis of dangerousness will reoffend
D.   Diagnosis is the strongest predictor
E.   Severity of the disorder is the strongest predictor

30.   In which one of the following situations you will not breach confidentiality of the patient?

A.   It is undesirable to seek patient's consent on medical grounds
B.   Information is required by law
C.   Next of kin requests for it
D.   For a research project with an approval from an ethics committee
E.   Benefits agency asks for it with a written consent from the patient

31.   Which one of the following is a stable dynamic risk factor associated with sexual offence recidivism?

A.   Lack of victim empathy
B.   Psychiatric illness
C.   Isolation
D.   Previous violent offending
E.   Depression

32.   What is the relative risk of psychosis in prisons?

A.   5
B.   10
C.   20
D.   30
E.   40

Chapter 8

Answers:
Forensic Psychiatry

1. D   Mostly perpetrator is a male. Indecent exposure can be categorised as Exhibitionist, Disinihibited and Aggressive, Impulsive and Antisocial. Exhibitionists usually don't have a psychiatric diagnosis where as the disinhibited ones are usually under the influence of alcohol, drugs or are having an acute onset of a mental illness or a relapse of a mental illness. However most of them don't reoffend. Rates of reoffending are; for first time offenders 20%, offenders with a history of sexual offence 60% and with a history of both sexual and non sexual offences 70%.

Incest is a criminal offence in which there is a sexual relationship between a man and a woman who are related as father-daughter, grandfather-granddaughter, brother-sister, mother-son and grandmother-grandson. If the female is above 16 years of age and consents to the intercourse it is still regarded as incest.

Chiswick & Cope: Seminars in Practical Forensic Psychiatry. (2001).

2. D   HCR-20 is empirically related to future violence. It is comprehensive and practically useful to generate informed team discussions to make decisions about management of violent offenders.

HCR-20 has been found to be a good predictor of violence and research supports its concurrent validity.

HCR-20 comprises of 10 static factors and 10 dynamic factors. The static factors are the ten historical items namely previous violence, young age at first violent incident, relationship instability, employment problems, substance use problems, major mental illness, psychopathy, early maladjustment, personality disorder and supervision failure. Whereas the ten dynamic factors comprise of five Clinical factors (lack of insight, negative attitudes, active symptoms of major mental illness, impulsivity and unresponsive to treatment) and five Risk management factors (plans lack feasibility, exposure to destabilizers, lack of personal support, non compliance with remediation attempts and stress).

HCR-20 should largely be seen as the first step in the risk assessment process. Although it is largely used in forensic in patient settings but it can be used in all clinical settings, however it may not yield accurate outcomes with all types of patients and under all manner of conditions. It should not be seen as a substitute for basic common sense and judgement.

Webster CD et al. HCR-20: Assessing Risk for Violence (Version 2) (HCR-20).

3. C Other factors include giving less emphasis to carers and members of publics' views, undue emphasis on civil liberties at the cost of increased risk, failure to properly implement mental health act and failure to share information in the best interest of patient.

Lipsedge, M. Psychiatry: reducing risk in clinical practice. In Clinical Risk Management (ed. C. Vincent) (1995).

4. A Only 10 of them had a diagnosis of schizophrenia and ever had contact with psychiatric services. However there are about 5000 suicides & 4000 deaths from road traffic accidents per year in the UK. Therefore risk of violence from mentally ill should be seen in perspective.

National Confidential Inquiry into Suicide & Homicide by People with Mental Illness: Safer Services (1999).

5. A Relational security has two components quantitative &

qualitative.

Quantitative is about, staff to patient ratio and amount of time spent in face to face contact, where as the qualitative component is about the balance between intrusiveness and openness; trust between patients and professionals. Therefore relational security is impaired by reduced continuity of care.

Kennedy H.G. Therapeutic uses of security: Mapping Forensic Mental Health Services by Stratifying Risk. APT (2002).

6. C   The degree of the restrictiveness of environment in management of a mentally disordered offender should be based on the clinical needs and risk assessment of each individual. Moreover restrictiveness makes a part of all three types of securities; Environmental, Relational and Procedural. Combination of all three types of securities based on risk assessment of an individual is called Therapeutic Security.

Kennedy H.G. Therapeutic uses of security: Mapping Forensic Mental Health Services by Stratifying Risk. APT (2002).

7. D   Legal communication is not monitored.

Procedural security includes policies and procedures which control access, communication, personal finances and possessions of patients. Within a service or an institution it also covers policies and practices in relation to quality and governance, including information management, legal obligations, audit, research and human resources. Specific aspect of procedural security include the management of violent incidents and acute excited states, including de-escalation, breakaway techniques, control and restraint, seclusion and forced medication.

Kennedy H.G. Therapeutic uses of security: Mapping Forensic Mental Health Services by Stratifying Risk. APT (2002).
Royal College of Psychiatrists. Strategies for the Management of Disturbed and Violent Patients in Psychiatric Units (Council Report

CR41) (1995).

8. E Stability has to be for at least one year however relapses may be abrupt, over days whereas for discharge into community from a low secure unit relapses should be predictable, taking place over weeks. With regards to a move from high secure to medium secure unit, stability has to be for at least two years.

Kennedy H.G. Therapeutic uses of security: Mapping Forensic Mental Health Services by Stratifying Risk. APT (2002).

9. E This issue remains under debate however it is clear that Black population is significantly overrepresented in both prison and psychiatric services. It has been argued that among British Psychiatrist race of a patient plays a role when clinical judgement is made. Moreover there have been studies supporting the notion that Black people are perceived to be more dangerous. It is however a fact that they have genetic predisposition to Schizophrenia, with it being diagnosed three times more frequently in Black people than in White population, but can this alone be a reason for their overrepresentation in both criminal justice system and psychiatric services (both secure and non secure). Further research is required in this area.

Riordan S. et al (2004) The imposition of restricted hospital orders: Potential effects of ethnic origin. International Journal of Law and Psychiatry.

10. C Adjustment of clozapine dose in this patient is important, since a substantially elevated clozapine concentration would otherwise be expected and toxicity may result. This is based on the fact that in smokers CYP1A2, which has a major contribution in clozapine metabolism, has increased activity, giving 1.5 fold less plasma levels in smokers. Caffeine has similar effect on the clozapine plasma levels.

Meyer JM (2001) Individual changes in clozapine levels after smoking cessation: results and a predictive model. J Clin Psychopharmacol.

11. D   All the antipsychotics listed in the question and in addition, quetiapine, zotepine and ziprasidone can be measured in plasma and reliable essays can be developed. However it is only clozapine which has substantial amount of data supporting a threshold target concentration (0.35 mg/L) associated with a good therapeutic response in many patients. Therapeutic range is between 0.35 mg/L and 0.6 mg/L as risk of convulsions is increased at trough plasma clozapine concentrations above 0.6 mg/L.

Flanagan & Spencer. Therapeutic monitoring of clozapine and norclozapine. CPMS Newsletter (1999).

12. D   There is no clear evidence that norclozapine is pharmacologically active in humans. Some early studies suggest that trough plasma clozapine + norclozapine concentration of 0.45mg/L is associated with good response in many patients. One reason for measuring norclozapine is that the result can sometimes give useful information even when the sample may have been collected before clozapine tissue distribution has been completed. In addition, norclozapine measurement in conjunction with plasma clozapine provides an index of clozapine N-demethylation, the primary reaction by which clozapine is metabolised. Saturation or inhibition of this reaction by co-administration of drugs such as fluvoxamine can lead to marked accumulation of clozapine i.e. clozapine:norclozapine ratio 2 or more. It can also give information on whether clozapine exposure was acute, chronic or acute-on-chronic. If the clozapine:norclozapine ratio is less than 0.5 or so one would suspect that no clozapine has been taken for some days beforehand, possibly a couple of days.

Flanagan & Spencer: A Practical Approach to the Therapeutic Monitoring of Clozapine.
Flanagan RJ et al (2003) Comparability of whole-blood and plasma

clozapine and norclozapine concentrations. British Journal of Clinical Pharmacology.

13. D   It is not a clinical term hence it is not recognised by either ICD-10 or DSM-IV. In accordance with Government's new legal framework dangerous people with severe personality disorder are to be kept in detention in specialist health facilities for 'as long as they pose a high risk to others'. The term DSPD refers to the following individuals:

A.   With significant disorder of personality.
B.   Who present significant risk of causing harm from which the victim would find it difficult or impossible to recover.
C.   In whom the risk presented appears to be functionally linked to the personality disorder.

Department of Health. Reforming The Mental Health Act. (2000).

14. A   Young males between 10 & 20 years of age account for approximately half of the recorded crime; the peak age of offending is between 14-17 years which is independent of any mental illness. One has to bear in mind that most psychotic patients are neither criminal nor violent and most criminals are not mentally ill. There is however a proven association of crime with youth.

Chiswick & Cope: Seminars in Practical Forensic Psychiatry (2001).

15. D   Only 17% of known offenders are women. 69% of female offenders are convicted of theft in comparison to 41% of male offenders. 19% of female offenders are put on probation in comparison to 10% of males. Women commit fewer serious and violent crimes.

Home Office. Gender and The Criminal Justice System. London: HMSO (1992).

16. B   In 63% of female homicides the offender has a psychiatric condition compared to 45% of male homicides. In depressive states the homicide may be a part of suicide pact with the victim, which the victim resisted. In men the conjunction of depression and homicide tends to occur in older age and most likely victim is the person's wife. Depression is recognised as a precipitant in homicides committed by people with unstable personality, in situations of domestic, social or financial stress. The most frequent primary mental disorder in homicides is personality disorder followed by schizophrenia and then affective disorders. Personality disorder is also the most common secondary diagnosis in homicides followed by substance misuse.

Department of Health. Safety First: Five-year report of the National Confidential Inquiry into Suicide and Homicide by Police with Mental Illness. (2001).

17. E This may be conscious act of punishment, or an unconscious displacement of hostility towards the husband. Of children killed less than 1 year of age 60% are killed by mothers. The two commonest groups of offenders who kill children are parents or parent substitutes (80%) and sexual offenders.

Palermo GB (2002) Murderous Parents. International Journal of Offender Therapy and Comparative Criminology, Vol. 46, No. 2, 123-143.

18. B It is also referred as to factitious illness by proxy. There are two components to the aspect of proxy: the creation of illness in another and the consequent distress caused by the doctor in the investigation of puzzling symptoms.
The perpetrator will frequently have had nursing experience and most common method used to harm is poisoning or suffocation. A common characteristic is that father is emotionally if not physically absent and is oblivious to the happenings.

Meadow, R. Fabricated or Induced Illness (Munchausen Syndrome by Proxy). In: ABC of Child Protection. Meadow et al (Editors) (2007).

19. A Profound character disorder, drug abuse and alcoholism are common among perpetrators of rape. Some perpetrators show evidence of intense homosexual fears, against which the rape may be seen as a defence and these may be experienced as at a near psychotic intensity.

20. E PPG measures penile tumescence. It has shown that some rapists are more likely than controls to be sexually aroused when shown images of rape. It is therefore potentially useful in the assessment of sex offenders and is also being used to monitor treatment progress of sex offenders at special hospitals. A positive result on PPG is an evidence of arousal to certain stimuli but does not predict future behaviour. False negatives may occur, for example, as a result of the wrong imagery being chosen, or by the individual successfully suppressing his responses.

Chiswick & Cope: Seminars in Practical Forensic Psychiatry (2001).

21. A Antilibidinal medication may be considered in some sex offenders but requires the patients' compliance and consent. Cyproterone acetate is an antilibidinal medication but is not a control drug. It works by reducing testosterone levels. Its possible side effects include loss of erection, gynaecomastia, inhibition of spermatogenesis, depression, asthenia, lassitude and weight changes.

Prentky RA. Arousal reduction in sexual offenders: A review of antiandrogen interventions. Sexual Abuse. Vol 9. (1997).

22. C Among patients with schizophrenia violence can take place in both acute and chronic phase of illness. They are over represented among the violent inpatient population. Acting on delusions is common in schizophrenia. Their victims are usually known to them and an attack on strangers is in fact a rare event. Substance misuse is usually a common contributing factor to violence in schizophrenia where as other contributing factors include situational factors, characteristics of the victim and individual's nature of illness (in terms of its phenomenology).

23. D Offending is less common in affective disorders than in other functional psychosis. Among affective disorders it is more common in mania and hypomania and may be serious. Violent offending is rare in depression but may be serious. Altruistic homicide happens in psychotic depression in this the individual has suicidal ideation which extends to killing his family to prevent them from facing the shame and stigma of a suicide in the family.

Chiswick & Cope: Seminars in Practical Forensic Psychiatry (2001).

24. C Schizophrenia can affect the risk of violent behaviour through three types of vulnerabilities; vulnerabilities that predate the onset of active symptoms which include developmental difficulties, dissocial traits, educational failure, increased rates of conduct disorder, non socialised delinquency and early onset substance misuse, vulnerabilities acquired as a result of active illness which include active symptoms, personality deterioration, social dislocation, substance misuse and unemployment, vulnerabilities imposed which include drug side effects (akathisia and neuroleptic induced deficit syndrome), increased isolation, erosion of social skills and incarceration.

Mullen, P. Schizophrenia and violence: from correlations to preventive strategies. APT (2006).

25. E Five main principles have been identified in the literature on offender treatment programmes namely; risk principle, needs principle, responsivity principle, professional discretion and programme integrity.

✐- **Risk principle:** the intensity of the treatment offered should be proportional to the risk of future serious offending.

- **Needs principle:** effective treatment targets criminogenic needs, that is, factor shown to predict future offending.
- **Responsivity principle:** the manner of the delivery of the programme should be consistent with the characteristics and abilities of the group being treated.
- **Professional discretion:** professional override is necessary in some treatment decisions.
- **Programme integrity:** the programme should be conducted in practice as intended in its theory and design.

Howells K et al. Challenges in the treatment of dangerous and severe personality disorder. APT (2007).

26. A   The forensic importance of morbid jealousy is its association with violence, often repeated violence, usually towards the sexual partner. Morbid jealousy contributes significantly to wife battering and homicides of spouse. The boundary between normal and pathological jealousy is indistinct, however frankly bizarre features like elaborate surveillance, delusional misperceptions or typical features of organic, schizophrenic or affective illness make the diagnosis very much easier. Jealousy may be psychotic or neurotic in type, or associated with personality disorder or substance misuse. Psychotic cases show a better response to treatment than others. It is essential to inform the potential victim of violence.

27. E   Instead it is 'understand the evidence'.
Fitness to plead should not be confused with fitness to appear in court, although some defendants unable to appear in court are also unfit to plead. Those unable to appear in court will include physically ill and some very psychotic defendants whose appearance in court will lead to a public scandal. It does not follow that a defendant who is highly abnormal and who does not act in his best interests is automatically unfit to plead.
The issue of fitness to plead will be decided by the judge not the jury. When the judge finds that the defendant is unfit to plead, the jury will decide whether the defendant

did the act or made the omission.

The Crown Prosecution Service. Criminal Procedure (Insanity and Unfitness to Plead) Act (1991).

28. B Almost every criminal offence requires mens rea or guilty mind. If the mind does not have ability to control physical acts, there is an absence of mens rea and this forms the basis of the defence of automatism. Legal definition of automatism has no relation to the clinical concept of automatic behaviour.
There are two types of automatism; sane (automatism simpliciter) and insane.

- **Sane automatism:** once only events due to an external cause. Examples include confusional states and concussion, reflex actions in response to bee sting, night terrors, dissociative states and hypoglycaemia.
- **Insane automatism:** the event is likely to recur and is due to an internal cause. Examples include epilepsy, sleep walking, brain tumors and brain diseases.

Chiswick & Cope: Seminars in Practical Forensic Psychiatry (2001).

29. C The best predictors of violence for the offenders with mental illness are the same as those for the ones who are not mentally ill whereas personality traits, diagnosis and severity of the disorder are the poorest predictors.

Monahan J. The prediction of violent behaviour: towards a second generation of theory and policy. AJP (1984).

30. C In addition to all the other options listed in the question, you can disclose information on grounds of 'in the interest of public' but this has to be an exceptional situation where the patient or someone else is at a high risk of serious harm. Otherwise a doctor must not disclose information about a patient to a third party which he has obtained from a patient in professional capacity even after the patient's death.

GMC. Confidentiality: protecting and providing information (2004).

31. A   Clinical stable dynamic risk factors associated with sexual offence recidivism include lack of victim empathy, cognitive distortions, low self esteem, anger, substance misuse, impulsivity and personality disorder. Whereas clinical acute dynamic risk factors associated with sexual offence recidivism include isolation, unemployment, deviant social influences, chaotic lifestyle, poor social support, affective disorders and substance misuse.

Craig LA et al (2005) Sexual recidivism: A review of static, dynamic and actuarial predictors. Journal of Sexual Aggression.

32. B   From a 5% sample of men serving prison sentences in the UK (Gunn 1991) identified a prevalence rate for inmates with schizophrenia of 1.2%.

The 1997 ONS Survey of Psychiatric Morbidity among Prisoners in England aged 16-64 years identified 10% of male remand, 7% of male sentenced, & 14% of female prisoners had a functional psychosis.

According to recent British surveys the prevalence of probable functional psychosis , adjusted for non-response and design clustering, was 4.5 per thousand (95% CI=3.1-5.8) in the household survey. In the prison survey, the adjusted rate was over 10 times greater: 52 per thousand (95% CI=45-60). Among male and female prisoners, rates were 50 (95% CI=42-57) and 110 (95% CI=100-120) per thousand, respectively.

Brugha T et al (2005) Psychosis in the Community and in Prisons: A Report From the British National Survey of Psychiatric Morbidity. Am J Psychiatry.

• ———— •

Chapter 9

Questions:
Addiction Psychiatry

1.   Which of the following is more specific for alcohol related liver damage?

A.   Gamma GT
B.   Carbohydrate Deficient Transferrin (CDT)
C.   MCV
D.   Creatinine Kinase
E.   MCHC

2.   What percentage of adults have lifetime experience of one illegal drug?

A.   15%
B.   23%
C.   28%
D.   33%
E.   40%

3.   In terms of Alcohol use which of the following statement is not true?

A.   In the UK roughly 93% of men drink alcohol
B.   In the UK roughly 70% of the women drink alcohol
C.   The distinction between normal and heavy drinker is arbitrary
D.   Greater number of alcohol-related problems occur in normal rather than heavy drinkers
E.   The term 'Alcoholic' is not used in DSM-IV or ICD-10

4.   It is believed that Alcohol has following effects on CNS except:

A.   Enhancement of GABA-A transmission
B.   Release of dopamine in mesolimbic system causing euphoriant effects
C.   Inhibition of NMDA-mediated glutaminergic trans-mission
D.   Amnesic effect through GABA-B transmission
E.   Ethyl alcohol is oxidised by alcohol dehydrogenise to acetaldehyde

5.   Heavy drinking (Alcohol) is more common in the following except:

A.   Men
B.   Lower socio-economic groups
C.   Those with lower educational levels
D.   Middle aged group
E.   Travelling salesmen

6.   Which of the following is a risk factor for Alcoholism?

A.   Family history of Schizophrenia
B.   Non alcoholic biological father but alcoholism in adoptive father.
C.   Alcoholism in identical twin
D.   Family history of Anxiety
E.   Young female

7.   Alcohol dependence syndrome described by Edwards and Gross constitute the following features except?

A.   Primacy of alcohol seeking behaviour
B.   Narrowing of repertoire
C.   Eye opener
D.   Loss of control of consumption
E.   Continued use despite negative consequences

8.   'Stages of Change' in terms of harmful patterns of drugs, as proposed by Prochaska and DiClemente include the following stages except:

A.   Pre-contemplation
B.   Contemplation
C.   Decision
D.   Action
E.   Outcome

9.   Which of the following statement about Delirium tremens is not true?

A.   Occurs in 2% of episodes of withdrawal
B.   Peak incidence is at 48 hours after the last drink
C.   Risk is increased by co-morbid infection
D.   Risk is increased by pre-existing liver damage
E.   Reported mortality is 5-10%

10.   Following are recognised neurological complications of alcohol abuse except:

A.   Auditory hallucinations in clear consciousness
B.   Extra-campine hallucinations
C.   Second person auditory hallucinations
D.   Marchiafava-Bignami disease
E.   Cerebellar degeneration

11.   Which of the following is not seen in Wernicke's encephalopathy?

A.   Lesions around the third ventricle
B.   Involvement of dorso-medial thalamus
C.   Lesions around aqueduct
D.   Degeneration of corpus callosum
E.   Involvement of mamillary bodies

12.   Which of the following drugs is not recommended

anymore during the acute phase of alcohol detoxification?

A.   Chlordiazepoxide
B.   Chlormethiazole
C.   Lorazepam
D.   Thiamine
E.   Phenytoin

13.   Which of the following statements about Disulfiram is not true?

A.   Disulfiram is also called Antabuse
B.   It blocks aldehyde dehydrogenise enzyme
C.   Causes extremely unpleasant side effects when used with alcohol
D.   It works as a negative reinforcer
E.   It involves restoring the normal N-methyl-D-aspartate receptor tone in glutamatergic systems

14.   A 27-year-old male was brought to A&E with complaints of nausea, vomiting and constipation. He developed respiratory depression and later he was also found to have osteomyelitis. Which drug could be responsible for this?

A.   Cannabis
B.   LSD
C.   Heroin
D.   MDMA
E.   GHB

15.   Which of the following drugs is most likely to cause tachycardia, arrhythmias, hyperpyrexia, irritability and tactile hallucinations?

A.   Heroin
B.   GHB
C.   LSD
D.   Amphetamines

E.   Cannabis

16.   Which of the following statements about cocaine is not
        true?

A.   Acts as a local anaesthetic at the mucous membrane
B.   Violence in cocaine users is common
C.   Carrying of weapons is more common in cocaine users
D.   Cocaine is associated with 'Crack babies'
E.   Violence and aggression does not show dose related
        association

17.   Home detoxification is contraindicated if:

A.   It's the first detoxification
B.   In patient service is available
C.   The craving is very severe
D.   History of fit within the last one year
E.   Previous unsuccessful detox

18.   Which of the following statement is true about a young
        female addicted to heroin?

A.   There is an increase in sexual activity
B.   She is likely to die of overdose
C.   Addiction is more severe than in males
D.   Is more resistant to treatment
E.   She is often a social rebel from a stable family

19.   A 19-year-old male is brought to A&E by police after a violent
        outburst. His parents inform that he has been becoming
        increasingly hostile for the last 2 month, which is unlike him.
        He is extremely anxious and irritable, and on physical
        examination he is found to have acne and gynaecomastia.
        Which of the following is likely to be responsible for this?

A.   Heroin
B.   Thyroxin
C.   Estrogens

D.   Testosterone
E.   Meperidine

20.   Acamprosite is suggested to reduce craving by:

A.   Blocking aldehyde dehydrogenise enzyme
B.   Antagonism of glutamate NMDA receptors
C.   Acting as negative reinforcer
D.   Agonist activity on dopamine receptors
E.   Inhibiting cholinergic transmission

21.   Which of the following statements is true regarding alcohol and driving?

A.   Alcohol misuse requires licence revocation until a minimum of 1 year of controlled drinking is attained
B.   Alcohol misuse requires licence revocation until a minimum of 1 year of abstinence is attained
C.   Alcohol dependency requires licence revocation until a period of 2 year free from alcohol problems has been attained
D.   Alcohol dependency requires licence revocation until a period of 2 year of total abstinence is attained
E.   Licence is revoked for a minimum of one year after single alcohol-related seizure

22.   The main psychoactive ingredient in cannabis is:

A.   Gamma- tetrahydro-cannabinol
B.   Delta-9-tetrahydro-cannabinol
C.   Delta-9-dihydro-cannabinol
D.   Delta-6-dihydro-cannabinol
E.   Gamma-9-dihydro-cannabinol

23.   Which of the following statements is true about cannabis?

A.   The onset of effects is usually within hours
B.   The effects usually last for 6-12 hours

C.　　The half life in body is roughly 80 hours
D.　　It is lipid soluble
E.　　Can be detected in urine for up to 2 weeks only

24.　　In terms of a relationship between cannabis and schizophrenia, the research in the last few years suggests that:

A.　　The relative risk of developing schizophrenia among high
consumers of cannabis use is 12
B.　　At the population level elimination of cannabis use is most
likely to reduce the incidence of schizophrenia by
approximately 8%
C.　　On an individual level, cannabis use confers an overall
fourfold increase in the relative risk for later schizophrenia
D.　　Cannabis has been found to be responsible directly as a
cause of death in patients with schizophrenia
E.　　Direct mechanism of cannabis, causing schizophrenia has
been identified

25.　　Drug screen remains positive for 2-5 days for which of the
following substances?

A.　　Amphetamines
B.　　Cocaine
C.　　Cannabis
D.　　Opiates
E.　　PCP

26.　　What blood alcohol level can cause death by respiratory
depression?

A.　　0.05%
B.　　0.1%
C.　　0.2%
D.　　0.3%
E.　　>0.5%

27.　　The number of deaths attributed to alcohol abuse each

year is:

A.   100,000
B.   200,000
C.   300,000
D.   400,000
E.   > 500,000

28.   A patient with a diagnosis of schizophrenia, who has been
       using antipsychotics for several years without any side
       effects, develops severe dystonic reaction. He had recently
       started using an illicit substance. Which is the most likely
       substance he is using?

A.   Cannabis
B.   Cocaine
C.   LSD
D.   Magic mushrooms
E.   MDMA

29.   Following are the names of some designer amphetamines
       except?

A.   MDMA
B.   MMDA
C.   DOM
D.   MOD
E.   Ecstasy

30.   A 25-year-old male describes having 'flashbacks'. Which
       of the following could be responsible for this?

A.   LSD
B.   Phencyclidine
C.   Cannabis
D.   SSRI
E.   Diazepam

.——————.

Chapter 10

Answers:
Addiction Psychiatry

1. B   Gamma GT (Sensitivity 20-90% and specificity 55-100%) and MCV (Sensitivity 20-50% and specificity 55-100%) both can be helpful but CDT is more specific and sensitive test. (Sensitivity 70% and specificity 95%).

2. D

3. B   In the UK roughly 93% of men and 87% of women use alcohol. The number of normal drinkers is far greater than heavy drinkers, which means that despite their lower rates of problems, greater number of alcohol-related problems occur in normal drinkers than heavy drinkers. The term alcoholic is used by Alcoholics Anonymous. ICD-10 uses the terms alcohol dependence and harmful use and DSM-IV uses the terms Alcohol dependence and abuse.

Semple D, Oxford handbook of Psychiatry 2005

4. D   Amnesic effects are through inhibition of NMDA-mediated glutaminergic transmission. Enhancement of GABA-A transmission produces anxiolytic effect.

5. D   It's more common in young people than middle aged. It's also more common in doctors.

6. C   Male sex is a risk factor, and history of alcoholism in blood relatives increases the risk (5 folds in first degree relatives). There is an association between psychiatric disorders like schizophrenia and alcoholism but family history of schizophrenia and anxiety is not a risk factor.

7. C   Eye opener is part of CAGE, a 4 item questionnaire used as a screen for alcohol problems. Alcohol dependence syndrome is a clinical syndrome first described by Edwards and Gross in 1976 though it is also often applied to the description of drug dependence as well. The features described form the core of both ICD-10 and DSM-IV descriptions.

The features include:

- Primacy of alcohol seeking behaviour
- Narrowing of repertoire
- Increased tolerance to the effects of alcohol
- Loss of control of consumption
- Signs of withdrawal on attempted abstinence
- Alcohol use to avoid development of withdrawal symptoms.
- Continued use despite negative consequences
- Rapid reinstatement of previous pattern of alcohol use after abstinence.

Edwards G and Gross MM 1976, Alcohol dependence: provisional description of a clinical syndrome. BMJ 1, 1058-61.

8. E   The 'Stages of Change' Model (SCM) was originally developed in the late 1970's and early 1980's by James Prochaska and Carlo DiClemente.

The SCM has been applied to a broad range of behaviours including weight loss, overcoming alcohol addiction, and drug problems among others.
The idea behind the SCM is that behaviour change does not happen in one step. Rather, people tend to progress through different stages on their way to finally making the change.

The stages of change are:

- Pre-contemplation (Not yet acknowledging that there is a problem behaviour that needs to be changed).
- Contemplation (Acknowledging that there is a problem but not yet ready or sure of wanting to make a change).
- Decision (Getting ready to change)
- Action (Changing behaviour)
- Maintenance (Maintaining the behaviour change), and
- Relapse (Returning to older behaviours and abandoning the new changes).

Prochaska JO & DiClemente 1986. Towards a comprehensive model of change.
Changing for Good, JO Prochaska, J Norcross & DiClimenteSep 1995, First Avon books.

9. A　　Occurs in 5% of episodes of withdrawal.

Delirium tremens (DT) is a potentially fatal form of alcohol withdrawal requiring inpatient medical treatment. It usually occurs in patients with alcohol dependence, who stop or significantly reduce alcohol intake. Onset can be within 1-7 days after the last drink though the peak incidence is at 48 hours. Risk is increased by severe dependence, co-morbid infection and pre-existing liver damage.

Symptoms include, acute confusional state, disorientation, amnesia for recent events, tremors, irritability, tachycardia, insomnia, nausea/vomiting (frequently secondary to gastritis or pancreatitis), hallucinations (auditory, visual, or olfactory), delusions, severe agitation, seizures, cardiovascular collapse, marked fluctuations in severity hour by hour.

Reported mortality is between 5-10%, though some even report up to 35% if not treated.

Management include inpatient medical care with i/v line access, isotonic saline, cardiac monitoring, oxygen, thiamine administration, i/v if necessary and benzodiazepines. Antipsychotics if hallucinations and delusions are not controlled with increased doses of benzodiazepines.

Wright T, Myrick H, Henderson S, Peters H, Malcolm R. Risk factors for delirium tremens: a retrospective chart review. Am J Addict. May-Jun 2006;15(3):213-9.

10. B   Second person auditory hallucinations are recognised form of alcoholic hallucinosis, there is some debate whether this is due to release of latent schizophrenia but the consensus favours the former. Other neurological complications include optic atrophy, peripheral neuropathies, central pontine myelinolysis, Wernicke's encephalopathy and Korsakoff's syndrome.

BMJ 2003, 183:304-313.

11. D   Degeneration of corpus callosum is seen in Marchiafavia-Bignami disease which causes seizures, inability to walk and dementia. Wernicke's encephalopathy is caused by thiamine deficiency usually related to drinking. If it is untreated it can be fatal.

12. B   Chlormethiazole is an effective drug and was used regularly in the past, but due to the risk of respiratory depression it is not recommended anymore. Although phenytoin is not used regularly but when fits are a complicating factor than it can be used before stopping alcohol.

13. E   This action is suggested for Acamprosite which works by reducing the craving for alcohol. Simultaneous use of Disulfirama and Acamprosite is shown to produce better long-term results in treating alcohol dependence.

Wilde et al, 1997.

14. C   Osteomyelitis is a complication seen in i/v heroin users. Other complications seen are local abscesses, cellulites and bacterial endocarditis as well as pulmonary oedema and coma.

15. D   Amphetamines can cause quasi psychotic symptoms

including auditory, visual and tactile hallucinations. Anxiety and depression is also associated with amphetamines. Intervention is harm reduction advice and there is no role for substitute prescribing in managing withdrawals.

16. E   Under controlled conditions violence and aggression has shown a dose related effect with increased cocaine administration (Licata 1993). Paranoia is more common in cocaine users and so is weapon carrying and violence.

17. D   Other indications for in-patient detox are history of delirium tremens, current confusion, co-morbid physical and mental disorder, suicide risk, severe nausea and vomiting, malnutrition and lack of stable home environment.

18. A

19. D   Anabolic steroids are widely abused by people for body building purposes and to improve athletic performances. Common symptoms are irritability, aggressiveness and hypomania/mania. Psychotic symptoms are also seen but less commonly.

Kaplan, 8/e, pp 454-455.

20. B   Acamprosite works by reducing craving for alcohol. The suggested mechanism of action is by functional antagonism of NMDA receptor. Its' shown to be effective as compared to placebo and clinically more effective in alcohol dependence when used with Disulfiram or psychosocial interventions.

Tempesta et al, 2000. Littleton 2007, Journal of addiction medicine 1(3) 115-125.

21. E   Alcohol misuse requires licence revocation until a minimum of 6 month period of controlled drinking or abstinence is attained. Alcohol dependency requires

licence revocation until a period of 1 year free from alcohol problems has been attained.

www.dvla.gov.uk, Gau S.S.F et al 2004 BJP 185: 422-428.

22. B

23. D   The onset of effects is usually with in minutes and lasts for 2-5 hours. The half life in the body is approximately 40 hours and it can be detected in urine for up to 3 weeks.

24. B   Latest research suggests that at the population level elimination of cannabis use is most likely to reduce the incidence of schizophrenia by approximately 8%. On an individual level, cannabis use confers an overall twofold increase in the relative risk for later schizophrenia. (Arseneault et al 2004). Andereasson et al 1987, found that the relative risk of developing schizophrenia among high consumers of cannabis use is 6. D and E are both false as there is no such evidence.

25. B   Amphetamines 1-3 days, cannabis 7-21 days, opiates 1-2 days, PCP 2-8 days.

26. E   Intoxication occurs at 0.1%, coma at 0.5% and blood level more than 0.5% can cause respiratory depression leading to death.

27. B

28. B   Cocaine lowers the threshold for dystonic reactions.

29. D

30. B   Phencyclidine is a hallucinogen also called PCP. In DSM-IV the term 'hallucinogen persistent perceptual disorder' is used for flashbacks.

.———.

Chapter 11

Questions:
Child and
Adolescent Psychiatry

1.   A seven years old boy presents with difficult behaviour and hyperactivity. Select one correct statement regarding Attention Deficit Hyperactivity Disorder (ADHD):

A.   Three core symptoms are-hyperactivity, no sense of danger and impulsivity

B.   Three core symptoms should be present before the age of 5 years

C.   Three core symptoms are-hyperactivity, inattention and impulsivity

D.   Incidence is estimated at 3-5% in the UK

E.   Methylphenidate is only used in ADHD children

2.   Mutations of Methyl-CP2-binding protein (MECP2) gene is associated with which of the following childhood psychiatric disorder?

A.   Conduct Disorder
B.   Rett's Syndrome
C.   Childhood psychosis
D.   Tourett's Syndrome
E.   ADHD

3.   A young child presents with obsessive behaviour. Select

one correct statement regarding Obsessive Compulsive Disorder (OCD):

A.   Childhood OCD has an earlier age of onset in girls than boys
B.   Pharmacological therapy is the treatment of choice in OCD
C.   In childhood OCD, obsessions and compulsions occur more commonly together than they do in adulthood
D.   It is a rare disorder in children and adolescents
E.   Clomipramine is less effective in treating OCD in childhood than adulthood

4.   Which class of drug would you use in a 9 years old boy with ADHD and Tourette's?

A.   Beta blocker
B.   CNS stimulant
C.   Selective noradrenaline reuptake inhibitor (SNRI)
D.   Centrally acting alpha agonist
E.   Selective serotonin reuptake inhibitor

5.   Which one of the feature is not associated with Gilles de la Tourette syndrome?

A.   Tics characteristically wax and wane
B.   Coprolalia
C.   Echopraxia
D.   Coprophagia
E.   A rare and bizarre syndrome

6.   Which is not true regarding risk factors in parent for physical abuse?

A.   Single parent
B.   Low expectations of child
C.   Child's physical disability
D.   Being Young as parent

E.   Mother's dysphoria

7.   All of the following symptoms are suggestive of autism
        except:

A.   Poor language development
B.   Poor or no eye contact
C.   Failure to establish friendships
D.   Stereotyped and repetitive use of language
E.   Extremely varied play

8.   How would you treat an intelligent 14 years old girl with
        moderate depression but no suicidal thoughts?

A.   SSRI and CBT
B.   SSRI alone
C.   CBT alone
D.   Tricyclic antidepressant and CBT
E.   Tricyclic antidepressant

9.   Which of the following feature is not associated with Fetal
        alcohol syndrome?

A.   It causes cardiac abnormalities
B.   Mental retardation
C.   Prenatal or postnatal height or weight (or both) at or below
        the 10th percentile.
D.   Included in ICD-10
E.   Down's syndrome is one of the differential diagnoses.

10.   All of the following are true regarding child sexual abuse
        except:

A.   It occurs among all ethnic, racial and socioeconomic
        groups.
B.   Girls are more likely to be abused outside of the family.
C.   Adolescents are offenders in 50% of the cases.
D.   The average age for first abuse is 9.9 years for boys and 9.6

years for girls.

E.   Children are most vulnerable between ages 8-12.

11.   Which is the first line of drug in an 8 year old with uncomplicated ADHD?

A.   Atomoxetine
B.   Metylphenidate
C.   Imipramine
D.   Clonidine
F.   Risperidone

12.   All of the following features are recognized in conduct disorder except:

A.   More common in large families
B.   Socialised and unsocialised conduct disorder is recognized by ICD-10
C.   Socialised conduct disorder is associated with normal peer relationship
D.   50% have specific reading retardation
E.   After the age of 18, a conduct disorder may develop into antisocial personality disorder

13.   A 10 years old girl cries and creates problems when goes to school. At home she is fine. What is the likely diagnosis?

A.   Conduct Disorder
B.   Depression
C.   Trauncy
D.   Oppositional Defiant Disorder
E.   School Refusal

14.   Choose one true statement regarding enuresis:

A.   Fluid restriction in a 7 years old boy with nocturnal enuresis
B.   Bedwetting occurs on most nights in 15% of five year olds

C. Secondary nocturnal enuresis is when a child has never developed complete night-time bladder control
D. Bedwetting may be related to a large bladder size
E. Treatment is not usually needed for children under nine

15. A 16 years old girl is diagnosed with schizophrenia. Parents ask you if there is any risk for her siblings to develop schizophrenia. What would be your answer?

A. 1%
B. 5%
C. 10%
D. 15%
E. 20%

16. A seven years old boy presents with behaviour problems. You note that he has small eyes, thin upper lip with smooth philtrum. Medical notes reveal that he has cardiac surgery when he was 3. Which is the likely substance mother might have abused during pregnancy?

A. Cocaine
B. Alcohol
C. Cannabis
D. LSD
E. Heroine

17. An 11 years old boy presents with motor and vocal tics. A diagnosis of Gilles de la Tourette syndrome was made. Which of the following will be the most appropriate treatment?

A. No treatment
B. Haloperidol
C. Fluexotine
D. Sertraline
E. CBT

18. Which of the following statements is not true regarding specific reading retardation?

A. Association with ADHD
B. An ICD-10 diagnosis.
C. More common in boys
D. An association with glue ear
E. All children have spelling difficulties

19. All of the following are true regarding Munchausen's syndrome by proxy except:

A. It is a form of child abuse
B. Mother is usually a perpetrator
C. More than one child may be involved
D. Mothers are cognitively impaired
E. Often considered as model parents

20. All of the following are true regarding psychosis in adolescents except:

A. Visual hallucinations are more common than adults
B. 80% of adolescents with first psychotic episode are admitted in adult psychiatric wards
C. Exaggeration of normal anxiety
D. Passivity phenomena is more common than adults
E. Thought disorder is not commonly seen

21. You are asked to see a 15 years old girl on paediatric ward. She is refusing treatment following a paracetamol overdose, despite high serum paracetamol levels. What will be the most appropriate action at this stage?

A. To use mental health act 1983
B. To use mental capacity act 2005
C. To ignore her wishes and treat on common law
D. Parents to give consent
E. To persuade her through family and friends

22. Which of the following features is usually not associated with Attention Deficit Hyperactivity Disorder (ADHD)?

A. Impulsivity
B. No sense of danger
C. Hard neurological signs
D. Symptoms before the age of 7
E. Poor attention and concentration

23. Childhood schizophrenia is associated with all of the following except:

A. Rare before puberty
B. Normal early development in most cases
C. Early presentation in girls than in boys
D. Worse prognosis than adult-onset schizophrenia patients
E. Inability to initiate plans

24. Common side effects of Methylphenidate includes all of the following except

A. Sleep disturbance
B. Loss of appetite
C. Dizziness
D. Tics
E. Heart palpitations

25. Effects of divorce/separation of parents on children include all of the following except:

A. Nearly half of all children in the UK see their parents divorce
B. Rejected and insecure
C. Boys adjust better to stepfathers than girls
D. Girls have more problems
E. Increased emotional and behavioural problems

26. ICD-10 criteria for anorexia nervosa include all of the

following except:

A.   Body weight is consistently 17.5% less (or lower) than that expected for height and age, or body mass index is 17.5 or less
B.   Distorted body image perception
C.   Amenorrhea in women, and loss of libido in men
D.   Weight loss is caused by the avoidance of foods perceived to be fattening
E.   Puberty in girls and boys may be delayed

27.   All of the following is true regarding cannabis use in adolescents except:

A.   Half of all 16 to 29 year olds try it at least once
B.   The plant is used as, the dried leaves- known as bhang, ganja, hashish, resin
C.   Cannabis can be detected in urine up to 56 days after it has last been used
D.   Children who use cannabis regularly have a significantly higher risk of depression
E.   Genetically vulnerable adolescents are more likely to develop schizophrenia if they use cannabis

28.   A poor outcome can be predicted for conduct disorder if all the following features are present except:

A.   Hyperactivity
B.   Early onset
C.   Greater total number of symptoms
D.   Aggressiveness
E.   Pervasiveness across situations

29.   All of the following statements are correct except:

A.   15% of all referrals to child psychiatric services are due to school refusal
B.   ICD-10 recognises reactive attachment disorder and

disinhibited attachment disorder
C. Children from small families are at low risk of psychiatric problems
D. Risperidone can be used in selected cases of ADHD
E. Sleep disorder normally peaks at 5-6 years of age

30. Children with IDDM may present with all of the following features except:

A. Acute ketoacidosis causing cognitive impairment
B. Conduct disorder
C. Generalized anxiety disorder
D. Major depressive episode
E. Acute Hypoglycaemia, associated with cognitive impairment

31. Which statement is true regarding atomoxatine?

A. It is a psychostimulant drug
B. It is a controlled drug
C. It is highly selective noradrenaline reuptake inhibitor (SNRI), which may be prescribed in children with ADHD
D. It causes deterioration in tics
E. It is specifically contraindicated to use with stimulant medication

32. Stealing among adolescent is associated with all of the following except:

A. Association with drug use and violent crime
B. Female problem gamblers are more likely than males to report psychological problems
C. Stealing behaviour reflects coercive and altruistic motives
D. Commonest antisocial act
E. Depression may be associated

33. All are true regarding depressive illness in adolescence except:

A.   Positive family history is unlikely
B.   Only fluoxetine can be given according to NICE guidelines
C.   Less psychomotor retardation
D.   ECT is contraindicated
E.   Promiscuity may be present

Chapter 12

Answers:
Child and
Adolescent Psychiatry

1. C   Hyperactivity, Inattention and Impulsivity are three core symptoms of ADHD. It is a persistent pattern of inattention and/or hyperactivity that is developmentally inappropriate. The behaviour should occur in atleast two settings (home, school or other) Incidence is estimated at 3-5%, in the USA (not in U.K, where the incidence is 1%). ADHD is highly co-morbid with 50-80% children having co-morbid disorder: specific learning disorder, conduct disorder, substance misuse, depression and anxiety disorder. Methylphenidate is pharmacological treatment of choice along with psychological and social interventions.

Applegate B et al. 1997 J Am Acad Child Adol Psychiatry.

2. B   Mutations of Methyl-CP2-binding protein (MECP2) gene is associated with Rett's Syndrome. A genetic disorder of arrested neurodevelopment that affects exclusively females.

Schneider JH and Glaze DG (2002) Pervasive developmental disorder: Rett's syndrome.

3. C   OCD is quite common in children and adolescents. Lifetime prevalence is 1.9% in adolescences. Cognitive Behaviour Therapy (CBT) is the treatment of first choice in OCD. Sertraline, an SSRI has a license for use in OCD from age 13 in the U.K. Clomipramine is significantly more effective in children with OCD and appears to be superior to other tri-cyclic antidepressants (TCA).

Rapoport JL, Inoff-Germain G (2000) J Child Psychol Psychiat.

4. C   Atomoxetine is highly selective noradrenaline reuptake inhibitor (SNRI) selectively blocking pre-synaptic noradrenaline reuptake transporter. It is now considered one of the first line of drug, prescribed in children with ADHD. It may be used in children with ADHD and comorbid Tourette's syndrome, as it does not deteriorate tics. It is not a controlled drug.

NICE Guidelines (2006) Use of methylphenidate, atomoxetine and dexamfetamine for attention deficit hyperactivity disorder (ADHD) in children and adolescents.

5. C   Coprophagia is the oral ingestion of faeces by the patient. Tourette syndrome is an inherited neurological disorder with onset in childhood, characterized by the presence of multiple physical (motor) tics and at least one vocal (phonic) tic. Tourette's is defined as part of a spectrum of tic disorders, which includes transient and chronic tics. The severity of the tics decreases for most children as they pass through adolescence, and extreme Tourette's in adulthood is a rarity.

Scahill L, Williams S, Schwab-Stone M, Applegate J, Leckman JF.(2006) Disruptive behaviour problems in a community sample of children with tic disorders. Adv Neurol. ;99:184-90.

6. B   Other risk factors are father's drinking, family's living in a community that is impoverished, history of abuse as a child and children's behaviour problems.

Cawson P, Wattam C, Brooker S & Kelly G (2000) Child maltreatment in the United Kingdom: a study of the prevalence of child abuse and neglect. London: NSPCC.

7. E   Rigid stereotype play is typical in autistic children. Autism is a pervasive developmental disorder that impairs social interaction and communication, and causes restricted and repetitive behaviour, all starting before a child is three years old. Most recent reviews estimate a prevalence of one to two cases per 1,000 people for autism, and about six per 1,000 for Autistic Spectrum Disorder (ASD).

Rutter M (2005) Incidence of autism spectrum disorders: changes over time and their meaning. Acta Paediatr 94 (1): 215.

8. C   A young adolescent with moderate to severe depression should be offered one of the following specific psychological therapies (for at least 3 months) as a first-line treatment:

-       Individual CBT, or
-       Interpersonal therapy, or
-       Shorter-term family therapy

If depression is unresponsive to psychological therapy after 46 sessions than a multidisciplinary review should carried out and to consider alternative or additional psychological therapies or offer/consider medication for young people aged 1218 years offer fluoxetine in addition to psychological therapy.

NICE (2005) CG28- Depression in children and young people: Quick reference guide.

9. E   Down's Syndrome is not included in the differential diagnosis. Aarskog syndrome, Williams syndrome, Noonan's syndrome, Dubowitz syndrome, Fetal Hydantoin syndrome and Fetal Valproate syndromes are considered in differential diagnosis.

Fetal Alcohol Syndrome (2004): Guidelines for Referral and Diagnosis. CDC.

10. B   Boys are more likely than girls to be abused outside of the family. Most children and adolescents are abused by

someone they know and trust.

Adams JA, (2004) Medical evaluation of suspected child sexual abuse. J Pediatr Adolesc Gynecol.17 (3): 191-7.

11. B   Methylphenidate is usually considered first line drug. National Institute of Health and Clinical Excellence (NICE) guidelines now recommend use of methylphenidate, atomoxetine and dexamfetamine as first line of pharmacological treatment.

NICE Guidelines (2006) Use of methylphenidate, atomoxetine and dexamfetamine for attention deficit hyperactivity disorder (ADHD) in children and adolescents.

12. D   1/3rd of patients with conduct disorder have specific reading retardation. It describes a pattern of repetitive behaviour where the rights of others or the social norms are violated.

Carr A. (ed.) (2000) What Works with Children and Adolescents? A Critical Review of Psychological Interventions with Children, Adolescents and their Families. London: Brunner-Routledge.

13. E   School refusal is a problem that is stressful for children, families, and school personnel. Failing to attend school has significant short- and long-term effects on children's social, emotional, and educational development. School refusal often is associated with comorbid psychiatric disorders such as anxiety and depression. It is important to identify problems early and provide appropriate interventions to prevent further difficulties. Assessment and management of school refusal require a collaborative approach that includes the General Practitioner, school staff, parents, and a mental health professional.

Fremont W P (2003) School Refusal in Children and Adolescents. Am Fam Physician 2003;68:1555-60,1563-4.
The Royal College of Psychiatrists-Factsheet 9: Children Who Do Not Go To School.

14. B It is primary nocturnal enuresis, when a child has never developed complete night-time bladder control. Bedwetting may be related to a small bladder size. Treatment is not usually needed for children under six, because in most children, it will resolve spontaneously.

Butler RJ, Golding J, Northstone K (2005) Nocturnal enuresis at 7.5 years old: prevalence and analysis of clinical signs. BJU Int (3):404-10.

15. C The risk of developing schizophrenia in general population is about 1% but it is increased in first degree of schizophrenic patients. Prevalence for siblings is estimated at 10% and life time prevalence for parents is 5.9%. The offspring of brothers/sisters of patients with schizophrenia have only a 2.6% risk for schizophrenia (on the average).

Goldner EM, Hsu L, Waraich P, Somers M (2002) Prevalence and incidence studies of schizophrenic disorders: a systematic review of the literature. Canadian Journal of Psychiatry, 47(9), 83343.

16. B Child has fetal alcohol syndrome. Fetal alcohol syndrome or FAS is a disorder of permanent birth defects that occurs in the offspring of women who drink alcohol during pregnancy. The following criteria must be fully met for an FAS diagnosis:

(1) Growth deficiency Prenatal or postnatal height or weight (or both) at or below the 10th percentile.

(2) FAS facial features All three FAS facial features present.

(3) Central nervous system damage Clinically significant structural, neurological, or functional impairment.

(4) Prenatal alcohol exposure Confirmed or Unknown prenatal alcohol exposure.

Astley, S.J. (2004). Diagnostic Guide for Fetal Alcohol Spectrum Disorders: The 4-Digit Diagnostic Code. Seattle: University of Washington.

17. B   Since the 1960's, haloperidol has been used for the treatment of Tourette syndrome (TS). Up to 80% of patients with TS initially benefit from haloperidol, sometimes dramatically. Pimozide and other neuroleptics can be used. Clonidine is also used by some.

Denckla MB (2006) Attention deficit hyperactivity disorder: the childhood co-morbidity that most influences the disability burden in Tourette syndrome. Adv Neurol. 99:1721.

18. B   ICD-10 has four categories of specific developmental disorder: specific developmental disorders of speech and language, specific developmental disorders of scholastic skills, specific developmental disorder of motor function, and mixed specific developmental disorder.

ICD-10 (1992) the International Statistical Classification of Diseases and Related Health Problems, WHO.

19. D   Mothers are not cognitively impaired or psychotic and often have a background in the medical field. There is no typical presentation for this condition. Suspicions may arise when parents misinterpret or exaggerate normal behaviors, and true cases range from apparent fabrication of reported symptoms to outright fabrication of signs of disease. Caregivers may report signs and symptoms that are undetectable to the medical observer, or the child may demonstrate signs that defy medical interpretation. The fabrication of an illness is a form of child abuse and not merely a mental health disorder, and there is a possibility of an extremely poor prognosis.

Schreier H (2002) Munchausen's by proxy defined. Pediatrics.110 :985 988.

20. D   Passivity and thought disorder are seen less commonly. According to royal college of psychiatrists report (a Scottish study), 80% of adolescents with first psychotic episode are admitted under adult mental services.

Boeing L, Murray V, Pelosi A, McCabe R, Blackwood D and Wrate R

(2007) Adolescent-onset psychosis: prevalence, needs and service provision. British Journal of Psychiatry, 198, 18-26.

21. E   Mental health act 1983 can be used only if there is mental illness. Mental capacity act 2005 is applicable only in people 16 or over. Parents have parental responsibility under children act 2004 and can give consent on her behalf, especially when she is refusing treatment. Any young person, under the age of 18 is considered a child according to children act. Common law can be used, if life is in danger and clinician can make the decision. When it is not life threatening situation, than involving the family and friends is often useful as they may be able to persuade the young person to give the consent, otherwise legal advice from trust lawyers should be sought.

22. C   Soft neurological signs such as poor balance and coordination difficulties are often associated. The term "hard neurological signs" points to behavioral signs that reflect brain injury, for example seizures, cerebral palsy, cranial nerve abnormalities leading to blindness and deafness and microcephaly.

Fellick et al (2001) Neurological soft signs in mainstream pupils Arch Dis Child. 85: 371-374.

23. C   Boys present earlier than girls. When childhood schizophrenia begins very early, the disease often manifests itself gradually and builds up to the first psychotic episode. Early signs of the disease may include social withdrawal, disruptive behaviours, academic problems, speech or language problems, or other developmental delays. These early signs aren't specific to childhood schizophrenia and may indicate a variety of other conditions. In adolescents, schizophrenia may also begin gradually, but the sudden appearance of psychotic symptoms and deterioration in hygiene and functioning is more common in this age group than in younger children.

24. E   Other common side effects are irritability, nervousness, stomach aches, headaches, dry mouth, blurry vision and nausea. Abnormal liver function, cerebral arteritis, leukopenia and death have been reported rarely.

25. D   Boys usually have more problems than girls. Emotional and behavioural problems in children are more common when their parents are fighting or splitting up.

Royal College of Psychiatrists (2004) Factsheet 14: Divorce or separation of parents - the impact on children and adolescents.

26. A   Body weight is consistently 15% less (or lower) than that expected for height and age, or body mass index is 17.5 or less. This can be due to either weight loss, or failure to gain weight during growth.

The ICD-10 (1992) Classification of Mental and Behavioural Disorders. World Health Organization, Geneva.

27. B   The plant is used as, the dried leaves- known as grass, marijuana, spliff, weed etc, and resin a brown/black lump, known as bhang, ganja, hashish, resin.

George C Patton et al.(2002) Cannabis use and mental health in young people: cohort study. BMJ, 325:1195-1198.

28. D   Aggressiveness alone is not a poor outcome factor provided if there are no difficulties in other areas.

29. A   5% of all referrals to child psychiatric services are due to school refusal and often associated with anxiety and misery.

30. A   Acute Ketoacidosis does not cause cognitive impairment.

Kovacs M, et als (1997) Psychiatric disorders in youths with IDDM: rates and risk factors. Diabetes care. 20(1): 36-44.

31. C   It is highly selective noradrenaline reuptake inhibitor (SNRI) selectively blocking pre-synaptic noradrenaline reuptake transporter. It may be prescribed in children with

ADHD. It is useful to use in children with ADHD and tics problem as it does not deteriorate tics. It is not a controlled drug.

32. B Male problem gamblers are more likely than females to report psychological problems. Stealing is most common antisocial act at all ages.

Shepherd J.P, Sutherland I, Newcombe R.G (2006) Relations between alcohol, violence and victimization in   adolescence. Journal of Adolescence, 29(4): 539-553.

33. D ECT is not contraindicated but rarely used.

Chapter 13

Questions:
Psychotherapy

1. Counselling does not commonly involve:

A. Dialogue between two people
B. Helping patients to find their own solutions
C. Guided advice by Counsellor
D. Exploring the past
E. Non judgemental reflection

2. How would you describe 'transference' to a patient?

A. Therapist's response to the patient's feelings and behaviour
B. Therapists empathy towards the patient
C. The feelings and patterns of behaviour in the patient, towards the therapist which unconsciously represent their earlier relationships in life
D. Process through which both patient and therapist express their feelings
E. Projection of undesirable feelings onto others

3. A patient with moderate depression is referred to you for assessment. Which of the following factors would make him suitable for brief psychodynamic therapy?

A. Being employed
B. He is less than 40 years old
C. There is a clearly defined psychodynamic focus

D.   Patient is keen to explore about himself
E.   Being highly intelligent

4.   Psychotherapy is usually contraindicated in:

A.   Normal grief reaction
B.   Abnormal grief reaction
C.   Psychotic symptoms
D.   Severe depression
E.   Substance misuse

5.   Which of he following is not recommended in behaviour therapy?

A.   Implosion
B.   Aversion therapy
C.   Covert sensitisation
D.   Systematic desensitisation
E.   Behaviour modification

6.   In the treatment of Personality disorder, a 'Step down' Specialist Psychosocial programme shows significant improvement in:

A.   Social adaptation
B.   Self harm
C.   Attempted suicide
D.   Re admission rates
E.   Personality

7.   Which of the following has shown to predict a good response in Psychodynamic therapy?

A.   Younger adults
B.   Intelligent patients
C.   Later alliance rather than early alliance
D.   Patient's perception of working alliance
E.   Therapist's perception of working alliance

8.   During a session of psychodynamic therapy a patient mentions, 'he abused his child' just towards the end of the session. What would be the most appropriate thing for you to do?

A.   End the session without saying anything to maintain the session boundaries
B.   Explain to him that everything said during therapy is confidential
C.   Terminate the session and inform the authorities
D.   Ask him what he means by 'he abused his child'
E.   Try to interpret your own feeling in light of counter transference

9.   Which of the following form of Psychotherapies borrows some techniques drawn from Zen Buddhism?

A.   Family Therapy
B.   Counselling
C.   Dialectical Behaviour Therapy
D.   Cognitive Behaviour Therapy
E.   Cognitive Analytical Therapy

10.   Patients are allowed to contact their therapist out of hours between sessions by telephone in:

A.   Dialectical behaviour Therapy
B.   Cognitive Behaviour Therapy
C.   Cognitive Analytical Therapy
D.   Family Therapy
E.   Psychodynamic Therapy

11.   Cognitive Analytic Therapy was introduced by:

A.   Freud
B.   Jung
C.   Marsha Linehan
D.   Bowlby

E.   Anthony Ryle

12.   The terms traps, dilemmas and snags are commonly used in:

A.   Cognitive Behaviour Therapy
B.   Cognitive Analytic Therapy
C.   Family Therapy
D.   Rational Emotive Therapy
E.   Dialectical behaviour Therapy

13.   Which of the following therapies typically focus on 'Role transitions'?

A.   Cognitive Analytic Therapy
B.   Rational Emotive Therapy
C.   Interpersonal Therapy
D.   Dialectical behaviour Therapy
E.   Cognitive Behaviour Therapy

14.   Interpersonal Therapy is not indicated in:

A.   Dysthymic disorder
B.   Substance misuse
C.   Bulimia Nervosa
D.   Mild depression
E.   Moderate depression

15.   EMDR is found to be useful in the treatment of:

A.   Abnormal grief reaction
B.   Phobias
C.   Chronic psychotic symptoms
D.   PTSD
E.   Anorexia nervosa

16.   In EMDR:

A.   The Subjective units of disturbance scale ranges from 0 to 10

B.   Delusions are challenged
C.   The treatment model is based on CBT
D.   Patient takes the lead
E.   Selective abstraction is addressed

17.   In Brief Psychotherapy:

A.   Patient is typically seen 5 days a week
B.   Usually deep personality deficits are addressed
C.   Counter transference should be ignored
D.   Goals are not specific
E.   Symptoms are usually clearly defined

18.   Which of the following statements about brief psychotherapy is not true?

A.   It's contraindicated in situational crisis
B.   Is directive
C.   Is useful when the patient was functioning well prior to their current symptoms or crisis
D.   Usually aims at resolving patients current conflicts
E.   Regression is encouraged

19.   Outpatient CBT:

A.   Is less effective than imipramine in moderate depression
B.   Is as effective as interpersonal therapy in treating depression
C.   Is as effective as lithium
D.   Is as effective as venlafaxine in severe depression
E.   Is less effective than DBT in treating depression

20.   CBT is contraindicated in:

A.   Personality disorder
B.   Substance abuse
C.   Chronic psychotic symptoms
D.   Learning disability

E.   Anorexia nervosa

21.   CBT in Older Adults:

A.   Is less effective in treating depression as compared to young adults
B.   Is indicated in vascular dementia
C.   Is also based on 'here and now' model so it does not refer to early life experiences
D.   Is proven to be equally effective in different subtypes of depression
E.   May involve other family members

22.   Cognitive behavioural techniques:

A.   Can be applied with patients suffering from dementia
B.   Cannot be used by therapists without full CBT training
C.   Are primarily aimed to enable patients with depression to think more positively
D.   Are contraindicated in Substance abuse
E.   Are used by health professional when trained CBT supervisor is not available

23.   During a therapy session when a 30 year old female is asked about her childhood abuse, she is unable to recall any of the memories of abuse. Which of the following process might be involved here?

A.   Regression
B.   Repression
C.   Forgetting
D.   Denial
E.   Distortion

24.   A 40 year male is very angry and has strong internal impulses to be violent. He decides to start taking karate classes to get rid of his aggression in a more acceptable way. His decision is a result of which of the following defence mechanisms?

A.   Compensation
B.   Repression
C.   Sublimation
D.   Displacement
E.   Rationalisation

25.   The reaction of the therapist towards the patient in response to patient's behaviour towards the therapist is called:

A.   Reaction formation
B.   Counter transference
C.   Compensation
D.   Displacement
E.   Altruism

26.   Which of the following statements about Client Centred Psychotherapy is not true?

A.   There are no specific indications for use of this therapy in clinical settings
B.   Limits are usually set on attitudes rather than behaviour
C.   The underlying philosophy of this therapy is that the solution to the problems lies with in the Patient
D.   Self actualisation is considered to be one of the main factors in Client centred therapy
E.   The therapist usually withholds giving advice or making interpretations

27.   The main therapeutic aims of long term supportive psychotherapy in treatment resistant psychosis does not include:

A.   Establishment of a therapeutic alliance.
B.   Promoting a better adaptation to reality
C.   Promoting awareness of transference issues

D.   Decreasing the reliance on medication in the long term
E.   Facilitating the maturation of defences

28.   The techniques involved in Dynamic Psychotherapy do
        not include:

A.   Free association
B.   Examination of Parapraxes
C.   Examination of dreams
D.   Acquisition
E.   Neutrality

29.   Which of the following statements is true regarding the
        initial appraisal, when an individual is faced with a
        potentially stressful event?

A.   The three secondary appraisal processes that individuals
        engage in when faced with potentially stressful events are
        threat, loss, and challenge
B.   Perception of the enormity of the threat being part of
        secondary appraisal
C.   Perception of the extent of the threat being part of primary
        appraisal
D.   Threat and loss in primary appraisals are found to be
        related to better psychological adjustment
E.   Challenge primary appraisals are found to be related to
        poorer psychological adjustment

30.   Factors that predict good outcome in Brief Dynamic
        Therapy include all of the following except:

A.   Evidence of achievement
B.   At least one good relationship
C.   Not chronically phobic
D.   Circumscribed problem
E.   Ability of the patient to express feelings at any stage

.———.

Chapter 14

Answers:
Psychotherpy

1. D   Counselling is a method of relieving distress by dialogue between two people and the aim is to help patient find their own solutions by giving support and appropriate advice involving non-judgemental reflection. Psychodynamic therapy usually involves exploring the past and although there is some overlap and it's also done in Counselling but not commonly.

Psychotherapy and Counselling in Practice. A Narrative Framework By Digby Tantam. Cambridge university press, 2002.

2. C

3. C

4. D   Psychotherapy is used in mild to moderate depression but not in severe depression. It's contraindicated in acute psychotic illness but can be used in chronic psychotic symptoms.

Semple D (2005)Oxford Handbook of Psychiatry.

5. B   Implosion, systematic desensitisation and behaviour modification are commonly used in behaviour therapy. Covert techniques are not very common but still used, for example antabuse in alcohol dependency. Aversion therapy, (Negative reinforcement) previously used to treat sexual deviancy is not recommended anymore for ethical reasons.

6. A   By 24 months, patients in the step-down condition showed significant improvements on all measures. Patients in the long-term residential model showed significant improvements in symptom severity, social adaptation, and global functioning, while no changes were achieved in self-harm, attempted suicide, and readmission rates. Patients in the general psychiatric group showed no improvement on any variables except self-harm and hospital readmissions.

Am J Psychiatry (2004) 161:1463-1470.

7. D   Early alliance in therapy rather than later alliance predicts good response. Therapist's perception also predicts good response but patient's perception has shown to be a better predictor of good response.

8. D   It's very important in therapy to maintain strict boundaries but always remember that safety of the patient and public triumphs everything else including confidentiality (Read Tarasoft case 1 and 2). Similarly understanding and interpretation of processes like transference is very important but safety comes first. You have to first clarify what he means by abuse before you take any drastic action like contacting the authorities. There could be many explanations for what he has said. For example he might be becoming psychotic and delusional.

9. C

10. A   DBT is mainly used for patients with Borderline Personality disorder. DBT can be described as a hybrid using Dialectical thinking and borrowing elements of CBT and Zen Buddhism. The treatment has a manual. It usually comprises of one-year programme in out patient settings including weekly individual sessions, attending weekly skills training group and out of hours telephone contact

and weekly consultation meeting for the therapy team. It is one of the few therapies with evidence base in the form of RCTs.

Robert L Palmer, APT 2002, vol 8, pp.10-16.

11. E

12. B   Anthony Ryle introduced Cognitive Analytic Therapy in 1990. It involves a therapist and a patient working together to look at what has hindered changes in the past, in order to understand better how to move forward in the present. Questions like 'Why do I always end up feeling like this?' become more answerable. It is designed to enable patients to gain an understanding of how the difficulties they experience may be made worse by their habitual coping mechanisms. Problems are understood in the light of patient's personal histories and life experiences. The focus is on recognising how these coping procedures originated and how they can be adapted and improved. Then, mobilising the patients' own strengths and resources, plans are developed to bring about change. It is usually time limited (12 16 sessions). It recognises maladaptive behaviours maintained by 'neurotic repetition'. The 3 essential patterns of neurotic repetition are 'Snags' 'Dilemmas' and 'Traps'. The technique involves '3 Rs', Recognition (of maladaptive behaviours and beliefs), Reformulation and Revision. In the end both therapist and patient write goodbye letters summarising progress and formally closing the relationship.

Ryle 1990 and 1995. Imelda Duigan & Susan Mitzman 1994. Www.acat.me.uk

13. C

14. B   Interpersonal Psychotherapy (IPT) is a time-limited psychotherapy that was initially developed in the 1970s by Klerman and Weissman as an outpatient treatment for adults with depression though it's now also used for disorders like Bulimia Nervosa, Dysthymic disorder and currently being tested for several other disorders. It is not indicated in treatment of substance misuse or as a monotherapy in severe depression or psychosis. Although IPT has its roots in psychodynamic theory, it takes its cues from contemporary cognitive behavioural approaches both in that it is time-limited and also in its use of homework, structured interviews and assessment tools. IPT is based on the belief that psychological problems are due to communication problems, which are formed due to attachment styles. The focuses of treatment are usually the current interpersonal relationships and their relationship to the development of illness.

Weissman, M.M.Markowitz, J.C., & Klerman, G.L. (2007). Clinician's quick guide to interpersonal psychotherapy. New York: Oxford University Press.

15. D

16. A Eye Movement Desensitization and Reprocessing (EMDR) integrates elements of many effective psychotherapies in structured protocols that are designed to maximize treatment effects. These include psychodynamic, cognitive behavioural, interpersonal, experiential, and body-centered therapies. EMDR is an information processing therapy and uses an eight phase approach. EMDR is said to eliminate or decrease emotional distress related to past memories, hence used in PTSD.

Shapiro, F. (2001). Eye Movement Desensitization and Reprocessing: Basic Principles, Protocols and Procedures (2nd ed.). New York: Guilford Press.

17. E

18. A Brief psychotherapy is short term usually less than 20 sessions. It is active, directive and used when the symptoms are clearly defined and specific goals can be identified. There are still difference of opinions about the effectiveness of brief psychotherapy, particularly the lastingness and depth of the results obtained, yet it is often highly beneficial, especially to previously well-functioning individuals who are involved in a situational crisis. Although probably the best results of brief psychotherapy are with disturbances of moderate severity and recent onset, in practice, it is often tried with a wide spectrum of patients. Brief psychotherapy aims at relief of the patient's major current conflicts rather than at change of his personality structure, which generally requires long-term treatment.

Primary Care Companion J Clin Psychiatry 2000; 2:1315, Pietro, Calif Med. 1967   September; 107(3): 263269.

19. B

20. D   CBT is one of the most commonly used forms of therapy and recommended by NICE for many conditions. CBT is an active treatment requiring patient understanding and engagement. Patient needs to be motivated and be able to link thought and emotions. It's main indications are mild to moderate depressive illness, Eating disorders (mainly Anorexia nervosa and Bulimia nervosa), Anxiety disorders and in selected patients it's also used in Personality disorder, Substance abuse and management of chronic psychotic symptoms. CBT is contraindicated in LD and Dementia, in addition to the general contraindications to psychotherapy.

Semple et al. Oxford Handbook of Psychiatry. 2005 p 787.

21. E   Family members can be useful as co-therapists especially in tackling relationship problems. It is equally effective in both age groups. CBT is contraindicated in dementia. Referring to early life experiences can be useful in formulation. Option D is false, as it's not yet proven.

Gatz et al 1998, Scogin & McElreath 1994.

22. A   Although Cognitive behavioural therapy is not indicated in dementia but Cognitive behavioural techniques can be helpful in dementia to reduce hopelessness in future. Can be used by untrained team members under supervision of trained therapist. Main aim is to identify negative thinking to reduce bias and logical errors. Can be used in selected patients with substance misuse.

23. B

24. C   The concept and understanding of different defence mechanisms is very crucial in psychotherapy. According to Freudian psychoanalytic theory, defence mechanisms are psychological strategies brought into play by individuals, groups and even nations to cope with reality and to maintain self-image. This can happen when the id impulses are in conflict with super ego. Healthy persons normally use different defences throughout life. An ego defence mechanism can becomes pathological when its persistent use leads to maladaptive behaviour. The purpose of the Ego Defence Mechanisms is to protect the mind/self/ego from anxiety, social sanctions with which one cannot cope with. Different definitions are used in literature but it's the concept that is important. Below are simple explanations of major ego defence mechanisms.

Repression:
Forgetting the painful memories or unacceptable impulses by putting them into the unconscious mind. This may cause a conflict within, and consequently distress and symptoms.

Regression:
Reverting to previous maturational level to cope with emotional stresses. For example a 30-year-old male starts behaving like a child.

Denial:
Refusing to accept the reality because it's too painful or contrary to your expectations. E.g. developing cancer, but denying it is there and refuse to go to the doctor.

Distortion:
Similar to denial. The person reshapes the reality, which is more acceptable rather than accepting the true version of reality.

Displacement:
Taking out impulses on a target where there is less emotional risk. E.g. hitting a wall instead of a person.

Intellectualisation:
avoiding unacceptable emotions by focusing on the intellectual aspects. E.g., focusing on the details of an accident as opposed to grief and loss of a relative.

Projection:
Reflecting own thoughts or behaviour on others. E.g., if a man is violent he may accuse others of being violent.

Projective identification:
Similar to Projection. The individual attributes his negative response to another as a justifiable response to the attitudes he perceives them having. It's a very useful therapeutic tool for therapists.

Reaction formation:
A person adopting behaviour that is just the opposite of an instinctual urge.

Rationalization:
Giving a socially acceptable reason for a behaviour that actually was an unacceptable behaviour. E.g., Hitting a person and saying that he is a bad man and deserves it.

Splitting:
Separating the good and bad aspects of a person to avoid the uncomfortable mixed feelings towards that person.

Turning against the self:
Resorting to self harm when having aggressive feelings towards other people.

Undoing:
carrying out an act, which has the effect of unconsciously cancelling out and unacceptable internal impulse. Seen commonly in OCD.

Sublimation:
The substitution of a socially more acceptable mode of expressing the unacceptable internal impulses. This is a very healthy and mature defence mechanism.

Altruism:
Providing constructive service to other people to gain personal pleasure and satisfaction.

Suppression:
Consciously pushing thoughts into the preconscious. E.g., Suppressing emotions to deal with the current situation and than later accepting your emotions.

Freud, A. (1937). The Ego and the Mechanisms of Defence. London: Hogarth Press and Institute of Psycho-Analysis. Cramer, P. (1991). The Development of Defence Mechanisms: Theory, Research, and Assessment. New York, Springer-Verlag.
Semple, D (2005) Oxford handbook of Psychiatry.

25. B The understanding and examination of transference and counter transference is an essential part of Dynamic Psychotherapy and helps in diagnostic formulation.

26. B Client-Centred Psychotherapy is a humanistic form of psychotherapy developed by Carl Rogers. The therapist is non-directive and reflective and does not interpret or advise except to encourage or clarify points. The main philosophy is that the solutions to the problems lie within the patients and they reach a decision through self-actualisation. There are no limits set on attitudes. Patient is allowed to express him or herself, no matter how awkward or absurd. If they feel like smashing the whole room, they are allowed to say that but not allowed acting on that.

Significant aspects of Client centred therapy, Carl Rogers.

27. D

Alan M & Susie V M. APT 2008, 14: 42-49.

28. D   Acquisition is used in classical conditioning. Other techniques used in Dynamic Psychotherapy are examination of the symbolism of neurotic symptoms, exploration of transference/counter transference and interpretation. Psychodynamic psychotherapy is a form of therapy, the primary focus of which is to reveal the unconscious content of a patients' psyche in an effort to alleviate psychic tension. In this way, it is similar to psychoanalysis; however, psychodynamic therapy tends to be briefer and less intensive than psychoanalysis, and also relies more on the interpersonal relationship between patient and therapist than do other forms. It involves gradual exploration of thoughts and conflicts in the unconscious to enable patient to understand their problems and bring about change by understanding, reflection and interpretation. It can be used in several conditions, mainly where emotional symptoms and behaviours can be understood in psychological terms for example personality disorders, mild to moderate depression and where there is significant impairment in social and interpersonal functions.

29. C   According to the theories of appraisal and coping, primary appraisals are concerned with how individuals evaluate the nature and meaning of a particular transaction (Lazarus & Smith, 1988), and Secondary appraisals, by which individuals determine what coping strategies are available to deal with a stressful event (Lazarus, 1966; Lazarus & Folkman, 1984). Three primary appraisal processes that individuals engage in when faced with potentially stressful events are threat, loss, and challenge. Typically, challenge is found to be related to better psychological adjustment, while threat and loss are found to be related to poorer psychological adjustment.

Ferguson, Matthews, & Cox, 1999.

30. E   Ability to express feelings at assessment is associated with good outcome. Other factors that predict good outcome include psychological mindedness, strong motivation, not actively abusing drugs, not chronically obsessed and being not grossly self destructive.

Jeremy Holmes, APT 1994, vol 1, p. 9-15.

.————.

Chapter 15

Questions:
Learning Disability

1. According to several well-constructed community-based population studies, what percent of children and adolescents with intellectual disabilities are likely to have a diagnosable psychiatric disorder?

    A. 15-20%
    B. 20-25%
    C. 25-30%
    D. 30-35%
    E. 35-40%

2. Social communication questionnaire has established validity for a diagnosis of which one of the following?

    A. Schizoid personality disorder
    B. Schizotypal personality disorder
    C. Autism
    D. ADHD
    E. Generalized Anxiety Disorder in Adults with learning difficulties.

3. What percentage of people with LD have active epilepsy?

    A. 15%
    B. 25%
    C. 40%
    D. 50%

E.   75%

4.   What is the rate of epilepsy among people with Down's
        syndrome who are over 40 yrs of age and also have
        Alzhiemer's Dementia?

A.   20%
B.   40%
C.   50%
D.   80%
E.   90%

5.   Which one of the following increases the risk of
        Alzeihmer's Disease in Down's syndrome?

A.   History of Alzeihmer' Disease in mother
B.   Smoking
C.   Aluminium exposure
D.   Baseline exaggeration
E.   Intellectual distortion

6.   A differential diagnosis of dementia in people with
        Down's syndrome who also have LD does not include
        which of the following?

A.   Depression
B.   Life events such a bereavement
C.   Hypothyroidism
D.   Sensory impairment
E.   Autism

7.   Which one of the following is not a feature of Klinefelter's
        syndrome?

A.   Hypogonadism
B.   Scant facial hair
C.   Shorter than average height
D.   Gynaecomastia

E.   Median IQ 90 with skewed distribution mostly in the range of 60 to 70.

8.   Which of the following is associated with tall stature?

A.   Prader Willi Syndrome
B.   Williams Syndrome
C.   XXY syndrome
D.   Foetal Alcohol Syndrome
E.   Cornelia De Lange Syndrome

9.   Which of the following is the most common feature of Williams Syndrome?

A.   Hypercalcaemia
B.   Sagging of skin
C.   Abnormal attachment behaviour
D.   Urinary tract abnormalities
E.   Supravalvular aortic stenosis

10.   75% deletion of paternally derived chromosome 15, in Prader-Willi Syndrome (PWS), is the complement of which of the following syndrome?

A.   Di George (Velo-Cardiofacial) syndrome
B.   Miller-Dieker syndrome
C.   Smith-Magenis Syndrome
D.   Angelman (Happy puppet) syndrome
E.   Williams Syndrome

11.   What degree of LD is usually present in tuberous sclerosis?

A.   Borderline intellectual functioning
B.   Mild
C.   Moderate
D.   Severe
E.   Profound

12.   Which one of the following Autosomal Recessive
        conditions is a preventable cause of severe LD?

A.   Phenylketonuria
B.   Sanfillipo disease
C.   Hurler Syndrome
D.   Laurence-Moon Syndrome
E.   Joubert Syndrome

13.   Which one of the following is the most common inherited
        cause of LD?

A.   Down's Syndrome
B.   Fragile X syndrome
C.   Tuberous sclerosis
D.   Klienfelter syndrome
E.   Di George Syndrome

14.   Which one of the following is not a feature of Martin-Bell
        syndrome?

A.   Large testicles and ears
B.   Long narrow face with under development of mid face
C.   Mitral valve stenosis
D.   Hyper extensible fingers
E.   Epilepsy

15.   Which one of the following is commonly associated with
        microcephaly?

A.   Down's syndrome
B.   Foetal alcohol syndrome
C.   Fragile X syndrome
D.   Hydrocephalus
E.   Soto's syndrome

16.   Which one of the following facial features described is not
        relevant to foetal alcohol syndrome?

A. Thin upper lip
B. Cleft palate
C. Small eye fissures
D. Big mandible
E. Joint deformities

17. Which one of the following almost exclusively affects girls?

A. Fragile X syndrome
B. Rett syndrome
C. Angelman syndrome
D. Klinefelter syndrome
E. Prader-willi syndrome

18. In a patient with LD, multiple changes in care staff and multiple short term residential placements are most likely to trigger which one of the following?

A. Depression
B. Anxiety
C. Behavioural disorder
D. Epilepsy
E. Sleep disorder

19. Brushfield's spots, low set ears, high arched palate, simian crease, syndactyly, protruding tongue and thyroid dysfunction are some of the clinical features for which one of the following?

A. Williams Syndrome
B. Smith-Mageris Syndrome
C. Prader-Willi Syndrome
D. Fragile X Syndrome
E. Down's Syndrome

20. Autism, ADHD and stereotypes like hand flapping represent a behavioural phenotype for which one of the

following?

A.   Williams Syndrome
B.   Smith-Mageris Syndrome
C.   Prader-Willi Syndrome
D.   Fragile X Syndrome
E.   Down's Syndrome

21.   OCD, multiple impulsive behaviour disorder including hyperphagia, aggression, skin picking represent a behavioural phenotype for which one of the following?

A.   Williams syndrome
B.   Smith-Mageris syndrome
C.   Prader-willi syndrome
D.   Fragile X syndrome
E.   Down's syndrome

22.   Severe ADHD, stereotypy's like self hugging, severe self injurious behaviour and insomnia represents a behavioural phenotype for which one of the following?

A.   Williams syndrome
B.   Smith-Magenis syndrome
C.   Prader-Willi syndrome
D.   Fragile X syndrome
E.   Down's syndrome

23.   Which one of the following is true with regards to sexual relationships for people with LD?

A.   They have no sex desire
B.   They have a normal sex desire
C.   They have increased libido
D.   Not even people with mild LD have the capability of being a successful parent
E.   They should not be allowed to get married

24.   For self injurious behaviour in people with LD which one
        of the following is a licensed drug?

A.   Risperidone
B.   Naltrexone
C.   Carbamazepine
D.   Lithium
E.   Fluoxetine

25.   Which of the following statement is true of psychotropic
        medications in the learning disability population?

A.   Ethosuxamide is a first line antiepileptic
B.   Lamotrigine has mood stabilising effects
C.   Valproate leads to weight loss
D.   Proprananol is an effective antimanic agent
E.   Naltrexone is an effective antidepressant

26.   In terms of psychiatric co-morbidities; depression, bipolar
        affective disorder, OCD, Tourette's disorder,
        schizophrenia and increased risk of autism are mostly
        associated with which one of the following?

A.   Williams Syndrome
B.   Smith-Magenis Syndrome
C.   Prader-Willi Syndrome
D.   Fragile X Syndrome
E.   Down's Syndrome

27.   Which one of the following is true for females with Down's
        syndrome?

A.   Delayed onset of menstruation
B.   Infertility
C.   Normal ovulation leading to follicular growth
D.   Delayed menopause
E.   None of the above

28.   What is the rate of successful control of epilepsy in patients
        with LD?

A.   30%
B.   40%
C.   50%
D.   60%
E.   70%

29.   Which one of the following is characterized by normal
        development until the age of 4 yrs followed by profound
        regression with disintegration of behaviour, loss of
        acquired language and other skills, impaired social
        relationships and stereotypies?

A.   Hunter Syndrome
B.   Rett Syndrome
C.   Phenylketonuria
D.   Disintegrative disorder
E.   Hurler syndrome

30.   Which one of the following has the highest rate of
        epilepsy?

A.   Down's Syndrome
B.   Fragile X Syndrome
C.   Angelman Syndrome
D.   Prader-Willi Syndrome
E.   Hunter Syndrome

31.   Which one of the following is true of offending in Learning
        Disability?

A.   Some evidence exists of increased rates of sexual offending
        and fire setting in the learning disabled
B.   Offending is more likely in severe learning disability
C.   Offences have no similarities with the offences committed
        by people without learning disability

D.   Offending has no association with any social disadvantage

E.   Learning disability together with schizoid personality features carries a high risk of offending

32.   Which one of. the following is true regarding psychotherapy in LD?

A.   Unmodified CBT can be used in severe LD

B.   Guiding mourning has no place in mild LD

C.   Progressive relaxation is part of psychodynamic group therapy

D.   Patients with severe LD who have been traumatized by abuse should have psychodynamic therapy

E.   Behaviour therapy should be used in groups in severe LD

.———.

Chapter 16

Answers:
Learning Disability

1. E   Co-morbid psychiatric conditions are more prevalent in learning disability population than in the general population. The common ones are schizophrenia, bipolar affective disorder, depression, ADHD, autistic spectrum disorders, obsessive-compulsive disorder, anxiety disorders, conduct disorder, tic disorders, and other stereotypic behaviours.

Schizophrenia may have a prevalence of 3% in individuals with learning disability, compared to 0.8% in the general population. Similarly bipolar affective disorder has a 2- to 3-fold greater prevalence in the learning disabled population than in the general population. Approximately 8-15% of children and 17-52% of adults with learning disability have ADHD and up to 15% require treatment for self injurious behaviour.

In the 1970 Isle of Wight study, as many as 30% of children with learning disability exhibited an emotional or behavioral disorder, compared to 6% of children in the general population. The study also showed that there was 56% risk of comorbid psychiatric illness in patients who also had epilepsy with learning disability.

Harum KH. Mental Retardation. eMedicine for WebMD (2006).

2. C   The Social and Communication Disorders Checklist is an effective parent-report measure for screening for pervasive developmental disorders. A self-rated version for adults has not yet been validated. It has an excellent sensitivity, but low specificity for diagnosing autism.

Skuse & Mandy. Measuring autistic traits: heritability, reliability and validity of the Social and Communication Disorders Checklist. BJP (2005).

3. B   According to a survey, 32% people with learning disability in an institution as compared to 22.1% people with learning disability in community had epilepsy, making epilepsy a common co-morbidity following psychological illnesses. In comparison, prevalence of epilepsy in the general population is between 0.4 and 1%.

Mariani et al (1993) Epilepsy in institutionalized patients with encephalopathy: Clinical aspects and nosological considerations. Am. J. Ment. Retardation.
Welsh Health Survey. (1995).   ·

4. D   Neuropathologically, Alzheimer-type abnormalities are demonstrated in patients with Down syndrome, both demented and non-demented and more than a half of patients with Down syndrome above 50 years of age develop Alzheimer's disease. Advanced Alzheimer's disease alone may be an important risk factor for new-onset seizures in older adults. Down syndrome patients aged over 45 years are significantly more likely to develop Alzheimer's disease than those less than 45 years and up to 84% demented individuals with Down syndrome develop seizures and the seizure type is usually of tonic clonic type. Late-onset epilepsy in Down syndrome is associated with Alzheimer's disease, while early-onset epilepsy is associated with an absence of dementia. In Alzheimer's disease patients with a younger age of dementia onset are particularly susceptible to seizures.

Down syndrome adults with epilepsy score significantly higher overall on the adaptive behaviour profile. Language function declines significantly more rapidly in Alzheimer's disease patients with seizures. In Down's syndrome there is a good correlation between the severity of EEG abnormalities and cognitive impairment, slowing of the dominant occipital rhythm is related to Alzheimer's disease.

Menéndez M. Review article. Down syndrome, Alzheimer's disease and seizures. Brain and Development (2005).

5. A It is thought that people with Down's syndrome who have Alzheimer's disease are similar to people with familial Alzheimer's disease, in that the onset of dementia is usually early. It should be noted that the mothers of individuals with Down's syndrome seem to have a specific vulnerability to developing Alzheimer's disease. Baseline exaggeration is exacerbation of cognitive deficits and maladaptive behaviours that pre-date the dementia. It can make determining the onset of dementia difficult in people with learning disabilities. Intellectual distortion (reduced abstraction) and often the reduced ability to communicate clearly can also lead to difficulty in identifying subjective symptoms.

Stanton & Coetzee. Down's syndrome and dementia. Advances in Psychiatric Treatment (2004).

6. E Autism or ASD comprise a spectrum of severe developmental and neuropsychiatric disorders that are usually apparent by the age of 3 yrs. On the other hand mean age of onset of dementia in Down's syndrome is in the early part of the fifth decade, characterised by impairment of higher cerebral functions including perception, memory, language, aphasia, agnosia and apraxia.

Bregman JD and Volkmer FR. Journal of Am Acad of Child and Adol (1998).

7. C They are taller than average, approximately 4 cm. Klinefelter Syndrome is a sex chromosome trisomy with a Karyotype of XXY; 1: 1000 male births (50% due to maternal and 50% due to paternal non dysjunction).

About 40% of patients have taurodontism, which is characterized by enlargement of the molar teeth by an extension of the pulp. The incidence rate is about 1% in healthy XY individuals.

8. C   XXY is a karyotype for Klinefelter syndrome which is associated with tall stature. All the other listed syndromes in the question are associated with short stature.

9. A   Williams syndrome is due to deletion on band 7q11.23 near the elastin gene.

The incidence of hypercalcaemia is approximately 50% therefore a diagnosis of Williams syndrome should be considered after an incidental finding of idiopathic hypercalcemia or a characteristic cardiac lesion such as supravalvular aortic stenosis. Other cardiac lesions in patients with Williams syndrome can include pulmonary stenosis and mitral valve regurgitation. Arterial hypertension may also be present.

Children with Williams syndrome are generally full-term infants. Microcephaly in one third of children and postnatal failure to thrive is typical.

Typical facial features include; "Elfin facies" - short upturned nose, flat nasal bridge, long philtrum, flat malar area, wide mouth, full lips, dental malocclusion and widely spaced teeth, micrognathia, stellate irides, and periorbital fullness. The voice may be harsh. Nails tend to be hypoplastic and the skin soft and lax. Ocular findings can include strabismus, a stellate iris, cataract, retinal vascular tortuosity, and reduced binocular vision.

Sensorineural hearing loss can be present and is likely to be under diagnosed. It can be aggravated by conductive loss due to middle ear effusions.

Behaviour phenotype for Williams syndrome presents as pseudo-mature language ability, initially affectionate and engaging, later anxious, hyperactive and uncooperative.

10. D   Main clinical features of Prader-Willi Syndrome (PWS)

include short stature, miropenis, cryptorchidism, behavioural disorders (over eating, obesity and self injurious behaviour), speech abnormalities and mild to moderate LD.

Angelman (Happy Puppet) syndrome is the complement of PWS as it is due to 80% deletion of maternally derived chromosome 15. About 90% of people with Angelman syndrome develop epilepsy.

The diagnosis of Angelman syndrome is based on history of delayed motor milestones especially speech, epilepsy, fine tremors, jerky limb movements, hand flapping and a wide based, stiff-legged gait and a happy disposition with frequent laughter.

All the other syndromes listed in the question are also due to deletions of chromosomes but the origin of the deleted chromosome is not from a specific parent.

Cassidy SB. Prader-Willi syndrome Journal of Med Genet (1997)
Williams CA et al. Angelman syndrome 2005: updated consensus for diagnostic criteria. Am J Med Genet (2006).

11.D They present with varying degree of LD (50%) but it is usually severe. 90% of tuberous sclerosis patients have seizures which usually take the form of "salaam attacks".

Semple et al: Oxford Handbook of Psychiatry (2005).

12. A In phenylketonuria there is deficiency of phenylalanine hydroxylase, leading to phenylalanaemia and Phenylketonuria. It is diagnosed postnatally by "Guthrie test". It is managed by supervised early dietary restriction of phenylalanine. Despite dietary treatment they have lower than average IQ.

Untreated children are normal at birth, but fail to attain early developmental milestones, develop microcephaly, and demonstrate progressive impairment of cerebral function.

Centerwall & Centerwall. The Discovery of Phenylketonuria: The Story of a Young Couple, Two Retarded Children, and a Scientist. Pediatrics (2000).

13. B   Fragile X syndrome is the most common inherited cause of LD affecting 1:4000 males and 1:8000 females with X-linked dominant transmission. Penetrance is low but greater in males than females, due to protective effects of second normal X chromosome in females. On the other hand Down's Syndrome is the most common genetic cause of LD. It is due to trisomy of chromosome 21.

Semple et al: Oxford Handbook of Psychiatry (2005).

14. C   They instead have mitral valve prolaps.
Fragile X syndrome is also called Martin-Bell syndrome and Escalante's syndrome. Its clinical features are macro-orchidism, prognathism, gynecomastia, hypotonia and autism, and a characteristic but variable face with large ears, long face, high-arched palate and malocclusion. Additional abnormalities may include lordosis, heart defect, pectus excavatum, flat feet, shortening of the tubular bones of the hands, and joint laxity. Females who have one fragile chromosome and one normal X chromosome may range from normal to mild manifestations of the fragile X syndrome.
Behavioral characteristics in Fragile X syndrome may include stereotypic movements (e.g., hand-flapping), ADHD and atypical social development, particularly shyness and limited eye contact.

Crawford et al. FMR1 and the Fragile X syndrome: Human genome epidemiology review. Genet Med.(2001).

15. B   Hydrocephalus and Fragile X syndrome have macrocephaly whereas Soto's syndrome has macrocrania.

16. D   Instead they have small maxillae and mandibles.
In foetal alcohol syndrome foetus of women who drink alcohol during pregnancy develop permanent birth

defects. It is not known whether amount, frequency or timing of alcohol consumption during pregnancy causes a difference in the degree of damage done to the foetus. Alcohol crosses the placental barrier and can stunt foetal growth create distinctive facial stigmata, damage neurons and brain structures, and cause other physical, mental, or behavioural problems.

Foetal alcohol exposure is the leading known cause of learning disability in the western world.

At the time of birth the foetus may show signs of alcohol withdrawal in the form of irritability, hypotonia, tremors or seizures). There are three distinctive and diagnostically significant facial features known to result from prenatal alcohol exposure and distinguishes foetal alcohol syndrome from other disorders with partially overlapping characteristics and may also be indicative of brain damage. The three facial features include a smooth philtrum, thin vermilion and small palpebral fissures. Other features in addition to the ones listed in the question are growth deficits and microcephaly, high incidence of mild LD, associated behavior problems, poor visual acuity, hearing loss, language deficits, atrial septal defect, ventricular septal defect, renal hypoplasia and bladder diverticuli.

Stratton et al. Fetal alcohol syndrome: diagnosis, epidemiology, prevention, and treatment. Institute of medicine (iom), washington, dc: national academy press (1996).

17. B   Rett syndrome is caused by sporadic mutations in the gene encoding methyl-CpG binding protein 2 (MeCP2) located on the X chromosome. It almost exclusively affects girls as male fetuses with the disorder rarely survive to term.

Incidence of Rett syndrome is 1:1000-15000. Clinical features include normal development up to 18-24 months followed by development of abnormal involuntary movements and often with autistic features. By age 5, 72% develop epilepsy (but eventually 90% develop epilepsy) and general progression is to spasticity of the limbs, eventually developing contractures and deformities. They can also have low mood, anxiety, sleep problems (involves laughing whilst asleep) and self injury behaviour. They develop moderate to severe LD.

Semple D, et al: Oxford Handbook of Psychiatry (2005)
Chahrour & Zoghbi. The Story of Rett Syndrome: From Clinic to Neurobiology. Neuron, vol 56 (2007).

18. C　　These are the most common precipitants of behavioural disorder. Therefore it is vital that any assessment for behavioural problems should include social relation, specific environmental stressors, consistency of care and lack of stimulation.

19. E　　Down's syndrome is the commonest genetic disorder caused by the presence of all or part of an extra 21st chromosome. Individuals with Down syndrome tend to have a lower than average cognitive ability, often ranging from mild to moderate learning disabilities. A small number have severe to profound mental disability. The incidence of Down syndrome is estimated at 1 per 800 to 1,000 births, although these statistics are heavily influenced by, in particular, the age of the mother. Other factors may also play a role. Individuals with Down syndrome may have some or all of the following physical characteristics: oblique eye fissures with epicanthic skin folds , muscle hypotonia, a flat nasal bridge, a single palmar crease, a protruding tongue, low set ears, a short neck, white spots on the iris known as Brushfield spots, excessive joint laxity including atlanto-axial instability, congenital heart defects, and a single flexion furrow of the fifth finger. In addition, individuals with Down syndrome can have serious abnormalities affecting any body system. They also may have a broad head and a very round face (Mongolism).

Roizen & Patterson. Down's syndrome. Lancet. (2003).

20. D

21. C   It is the complement of Angelman syndrome with 75% deletion of paternally derived chromosome 15. The incidence of Prader-willi syndrome is between 1 in 12,000 and 1 in 15,000 live births.

Prader-willi syndrome is characterized by hyperphagia and food preoccupations, as well as small stature and learning difficulties.

Traditionally, Prader-willi syndrome was diagnosed by clinical presentation. Currently, the syndrome is diagnosed through genetic testing; testing is recommended for newborns with pronounced hypotonia (floppiness). Early diagnosis of Prader-willi syndrome allows for early intervention as well as the early prescription of growth hormone. Daily recombinant growth hormone (GH) injections are indicated for children with Prader-willi syndrome. GH supports linear growth and increased muscle mass, and may lessen food preoccupation and weight gain.

Cassidy S.B. Prader Willi Syndrome. Journal of Medical Genetics (1997).

22. B   Smith-Magenis syndrome is a developmental disorder that affects many parts of the body. The major features of this condition include mild to moderate learning disability, distinctive facial features, sleep disturbances and behavioural problems. It affects an estimated 1 in 25000 individuals. The syndrome is due to an abnormality in the short (p) arm of chromosome 17 and is sometimes called the 17 p syndrome.

Most children with Smith-Magenis syndrome have a broad, square-shapd face with deep-set eyes, full cheeks, and a prominent lower jaw. The middle of the face and the bridge of the nose often appear flattened. The mouth tends to turn downward with a full, outward-curving upper lip. These facial differences can be subtle in early childhood, but they typically become coarser and more distinctive in later childhood and adulthood. They may also have reduced sensitivity to pain and temperature, and a hoarse voice. Some people with this disorder have ear abnormalities that lead to hearing loss. Affected individuals may have eye abnormalities that cause myopia, strabismus, and other problems with vision. Heart and kidney defects also have been reported in people with Smith-Magenis syndrome, though they are less common.

Disrupted sleep patterns are characteristic of Smith-Magenis syndrome, typically beginning early in life. Affected people may be very sleepy during the day, but have trouble falling asleep and awaken several times each night, due to an inverted circadian rhythm of melatonin.

People with Smith-Magenis syndrome have engaging personalities, but most also have behavioral problems. These include frequent temper tantrums and outbursts, aggression, anxiety, impulsiveness, and difficulty paying attention. Self-injury, including biting, hitting, head banging, and skin picking, is very common. Repetitive self-hugging is a behavioral trait that may be unique to Smith-Magenis syndrome. People with this condition also compulsively lick their fingers and flip pages of books and magazines (a behavior known as "lick and flip").

Girirajan et al. Genotype-phenotype correlation in Smith-Magenis syndrome: evidence that multiple genes in 17p11.2 contribute to the clinical spectrum. Genet Med (2006).

23. B   Issues raised by appropriate sexual relationships will include consideration of contraception, understanding of the responsibilities of parenthood, issues of commitment and marriage. Many people with mild LD are capable of being successful parents.

Semple et al: Oxford Handbook of Psychiatry (2005).

24. D   Lithium is the only drug licensed for self injurious behaviour.

The Maudsley prescribing guidelines (2007).

25. B   Ethosuxamide is second line treatment for Absence seizures. Valproate leads to weight gain in 50% of patients. Several small studies have suggested that high dose propranolol has antimanic effect but there is not enough data to support its use.

(Bhaumik & Branford. The Frith prescribing guidelines for Adults with LD. Leicestershire Partnership NHS Trust. 2005).

26. E   18% of children and 30% of adults with Down's Syndrome have psychiatric co-morbidity.

27. E   Normal onset of menstruation, problems with ovulation and follicular growth and early menopause.

Semple et al: Oxford Handbook of Psychiatry (2005).

28. E

29. D   Disintegrative disorder (Heller's Syndrome) has unknown aetiology but may follow minor illness or viral encephalitis.
The condition develops in children who have previously seemed perfectly normal. Typically language, interest in the social environment, and often toileting and self-care abilities are lost, and there may be a general loss of interest in the environment. Clinically the child usually appears autistic but the history is not suggestive of autism.

Malhotra S & Gupta N. Childhood disintegrative disorder. Journal of Autism and Developmental Disorders (1999).

30. C   Both Angelman and Rett syndrome have the highest rate of epilepsy i.e 90%.

Semple et al: Oxford Handbook of Psychiatry (2005).

31. A   Offending is more likely in mild and moderate learning disability than in severe learning disability. It is more likely in association with family, social, and environmental disadvantages. Offences are broadly similar to the offences committed by the offenders without learning disability. Learning disability together with antisocial personality features carries a high risk of offending.

Chiswick & Cope: Seminars in Practical Forensic Psychiatry (2001).

32. E   Modified CBT and guided mourning can be used in patients with LD. There is little evidence for psychodynamic psychotherapy in patients with severe LD. Progressive muscle relaxation is part of behaviour therapy.

The rationale behind a group therapy is that people who mainly encounter problems in group settings can best be helped in group therapy. For severe learning disabled adolescents groups can be powerful. It can help them in their search for a healthier way of relating to others and help to develop both the confidence and the skills for interacting with others.

Nicholls T. 'Could I Play a Different Role?' Group Music Therapy with Severely Learning Disabled Adolescents. In: Music Therapy and Group Work: Sound Company. Davies & Richards (Editors) (2002).

•———•

Chapter 17

Questions:
Old Age Psychiatry

1.   Which of the following statements about Semantic
        Dementia is not true?

A.   Semantic dementia is a form of Fronto-temporal dementia
B.   It affects anterior temporal lobes
C.   Memory is preserved for remote events like Alzheimer's
        disease (AD)
D.   Onset is usually between 50- 65 years of age
E.   Orientation to time and place are preserved

2.   Which one of the following conditions is not associated
        with Neurofibrillary tangles (NFT's)?

A.   Alzheimer's disease
B.   Normal aging
C.   Semantic dementia
D.   Creutzfeldt-Jakob disease
E.   Supranuclear Palsy

3.   Which of the following statements regarding
        Cholinesterase inhibitors is not true?

A.   Rivastigmine is a reversible inhibitor of Acetylcho-
        linesterase (AchE)
B.   Donepezil, Rivastigmine and Galantamine are used in the
        treatment of mild-moderate AD
C.   Side effects are due to peripheral action of the drugs

D.   Galantamine prevents the breakdown of acetylcholine by inhibiting acetylcholinesterase (AchE) and butylcholinesterase (BuChE)

E.   Common side effects are GIT disturbance

4.   A 66 years old ex-smoker presents with cognitive impairment. Diagnosis of Vascular Dementia (VaD) is suspected. Which of the following statement is not correct?

A.   2nd most common cause of dementia after Alzheimer's disease (AD)

B.   Males are more likely to have VaD than women

C.   In most cases, autosomal dominant mode of inheritance is seen

D.   Abrupt onset

E.   Stepwise deterioration

5.   Which one of the statement is not true about Hachinski Ischaemic score (HIS)?

A.   Abrupt onset is one of the components

B.   HIS is based on 15 clinical features

C.   A score of 7 or more is indicative of Vascular Dementia (VaD)

D.   History of hypertension, depression and strokes are components of HIS

E.   A score of 4 or less is suggestive of Alzheimer's disease (AD)

6.   All of the following are considered risk factors for Alzheimer's disease (AD) except:

A.   Advancing age

B.   Down's syndrome

C.   Fish consumption

D.   Apolipoprotein E genotype

E.   Poor cardiovascular health (including diabetes, hypertension, high cholesterol and strokes)

7.   All are true about Apolipoprotein E gene except:

A.   It is associated with chromosome 19
B.   There are three alleles
C.   It is associated with early onset Alzheimer's disease (AD)
D.   Individuals homozygous for ε4 (ε4/ ε4) have a higher risk
        of developing AD
E.   ε4 is the rarest form in the general population but is
        commonest in those with Alzheimer's disease (AD)

8.   Factors associated with diminished survival in patients
        with Alzheimer's disease (AD) include all of the following
        except:

A.   Male gender
B.   Absence of misidentification phenomena
C.   Congestive cardiac failure
D.   Temporal lobe damage
E.   Onset <65

9.   Which statement is not correct about Dementia of Lewy
        Body Type (DLB)?

A.   Cholinergic deficit is more marked than Alzheimer's
        disease
B.   Dementia with Lewy Bodies is not a DSM-IV recognized
        diagnosis
C.   Short term memory loss is characteristic feature in the
        early disease
D.   Preservation of medial temporal lobes on CT / MRI scans
E.   Fluctuation in cognition

10.   All of the following statements are true about depression
        in elderly except:

A.   It is more common in men.
B.   Sensory impairment is a risk factor
C.   Suicide rates are higher in the elderly than other age

groups

D.   Organic factors can lead to depressive symptoms

E.   Delusions may be associated

11.   The clinical features of Alzheimer's disease (AD) consist of:

A.   Amnesia, aphasia, aprexia and agnosia (the 4 As)

B.   It is easy to distinguish from normal aging

C.   Amnesia, aphasia, agraphia and agnosia (the 4 As)

D.   40% of patients suffer with thought disorder

E.   Rapid onset

12.   All are true regarding Testamentary Capacity except:

A.   It is the ability to make a valid will

B.   There are five legal criteria for determining testamentary capacity

C.   The test generally requires that the testator is aware of the extent and value of their property

D.   Testator must know the names of close relatives and beneficiaries and be able to assess their claims to his/her property

E.   Testator must not be acting on delusional ideas

13.   Which of the following statements regarding Normal Pressure Hydrocephalus (NPH) is not correct?

A.   1-2 % of dementia cases present with Normal Pressure Hydrocephalus (NPH)

B.   It presents with cognitive impairment, gait disturbance and incontinence

C.   80% of patients with NPH are over 70 years of age

D.   CT scan shows periventricular hypodensities and normal ventricles with small sulci

E.   Dementia is predominantly frontal lobe in nature, with apathy, dullness in thinking, and slight inattention

14.   Late-onset Huntington's disease may present with all of the following except:

A.   Usually associated with milder disease
B.   Levodopa responsive parkinsonism is common
C.   Cardiovascular dysautonomia
D.   A preponderance of maternal transmission is noted in late-onset Huntington's disease
E.   Slow progression of symptoms

15.   Ganser Syndrome may present with all of the following except:

A.   DSM-IV classifies Ganser syndrome as a dissociative disorder
B.   It is very rarely associated with head injury
C.   Approximate answers
D.   Clouding of consciousness
E.   Temporal lobe epilepsy may be included in differential diagnosis

16.   Which one of the statements is not correct regarding prevalence of neurotic disorders in elderly?

A.   Simple phobia-4%
B.   Social phobia-1%
C.   OCD-3-4%
D.   Agarophobia-1.4-7%
E.   Generalized Anxiety Disorder-4%

17.   Which of the following feature cannot differentiate between Vascular dementia (VaD) abd Alzheimer's disease (AD)?

A.   Personality and insight are relatively preserved in VaD than AD in the early disease
B.   Patients with VaD are more likely to have emotional labiality than AD
C.   The fluctuating course of VaD helps to differentiate it from AD

D.   Presence of apraxia is suggestive of VaD than AD
E.   The Hachiniski score can not differentiate AD from mixed
       vascular and Alzheimer's disease

18.   Which of the following feature is not recognised in frontal-
       lobe syndrome?

A.   Epilepsy
B.   Over talkativeness
C.   Euphoria
D.   Receptive dysphasia
E.   Perseveration

19.   All of the following features are characteristic features of
       Delirium Tremens except:

A.   Visual illusions
B.   Olfactory illusions
C.   Clouding of consciousness
D.   Lilliputian hallucinations
E.   Severe autonomic instability

20.   All of the following are recognized features of Pick's
       disease except:

A.   Apathy
B.   General euphoria
C.   A frequently abnormal EEG
D.   Fatuous mood
E.   Intellectual decline

21.   Which one of the following statement is not associated
       with Sub-cortical dementia?

A.   Parkinson's disease
B.   Huntington's chorea
C.   Apathy
D.   Creutzfeldt-Jakob disease

E.   AIDS Complex dementia

22.   The following features are suggestive of temporal lobe lesions except:

A.   Contralateral hemiparesis
B.   Gerstmann's syndrome
C.   Contralateral upper quadrantic visual field lesion
D.   Prosopagnosia
E.   Prosody

23.   Which statement is true regarding functional psychosis in elderly?

A.   It has a prevalence of 1%
B.   First rank symptoms are present in 70% of patients
C.   Strong association with visual impairment
D.   10% have premorbid paranoid traits
E.   More common in males

24.   One of the following statements is not correct regarding affective disorders in elderly?

A.   More common in females
B.   A positive family history is less common
C.   30% of all cases of major depression occur in elderly
D.   Strong association with physical illness
E.   High prevalence in elderly nursing home residents

25.   All are recognised features of vitamin B12 deficiency except:
A.   Alzheimer's Dementia
B.   Paranoid state
C.   Depression
D.   Numbness
E.   Confusion

26.   All are recognised features of Non-Dominant Parietal

Lobe lesions except:

A. Autotopagnosia
B. Neglect of contralateral limb
C. Deficits in visual memory
D. Dressing apraxia
E. Constructional apraxia

27. Which one of the following definitions is not correct?

A. Constructional apraxia inability to draw shapes or to construct figures/patterns or to copy designs such as interlocking pentagons
B. Dysgraphaesthesia - inability to recognize letters or numbers written on the hand
C. Expressive aphasia Patient can not understand the spoken or written word
D. Astereognosia - Inability to identify objects by palpation
E. Asomatognosia Patient is unable to recognize parts of his or her body

28. The following features are suggestive of dysmnesic syndrome except:

A. Ataxia
B. Paranoid delusions
C. Recent memory impairment
D. Peripheral neuropathy
E. Confabulation

29. Recognized features of Klüver-Bucy syndrome include all of the following except:

A. Hypersexuality
B. Memory impairment
C. Extensive bilateral temporal damage
D. Visual agnosia
E. Extreme fear

30.   Risk factors for suicide in elderly include all of the following except:

A.   Alcohol misuse
B.   Female gender
C.   Physical illness
D.   Anankastic and anxious personality traits
E.   Single/separated/widowed/divorced

31.   82 years lady with dementia is admitted with Femur's neck fracture. What are the risks of her developing delirium postoperatively?

A.   15%
B.   25%
C.   50%
D.   75%
F.   90%

32.   Which antipsychotic is contraindicated in patients with dementia and psychosis?

A.   Haloperidol
B.   Olanzapine
C.   Quetiapine
D.   Chlorpromazine
E.   Sulpiride

33.   78 years old lady admitted to a general hospital being severely unwell. 5 days later, she began complaining to her daughter that staff are not treating her well and poisoning her food. What is the likely diagnosis in this case?

A.   Delirium
B.   Delusional disorder
C.   Psychotic episode
D.   Dementia
E.   Depression

Chapter 18

Answers:
Old Age Psychiatry

1. C   Semantic dementia (SD) is a progressive neuro-degenerative disorder characterized by loss of semantic memory in both the verbal and non-verbal domains. The most common presenting symptoms are in the verbal domain (with loss of word meaning) and it is therefore often characterized (incorrectly) as a primary language disorder (a so-called progressive fluent aphasia). Clinical signs include fluent aphasia, anomia, impaired comprehension of word meaning, and visual associative agnosia. Memory is better for recent rather than for remote events (unlike AD).

Neary D et als. (1998) Frontotemporal lobar degeneration: a consensus on clinical diagnostic criteria." 'Neurology' 51(6):1546-54.

2. C   Semantic dementia is not associated. Neurofibrillary tangles are pathological protein aggregates found within neurons in cases of Alzheimer's disease. Tangles are formed by hyperphosphorylation of a microtubule-associated protein known as tau, causing it to aggregate in an insoluble form. NFT's are found in the dysrrophic neuritis of plaques.

Conrad C, Andreadis A, Trojanowski JQ, et als (1997) Genetic Evidence For the Involvement of Tau In Progressive Supranuclear Palsy. Annals of Neurology 41: 277-281.

3. A -   An acetylcholinesterase inhibitor or anti-cholinesterase is a chemical that inhibits the cholinesterase enzyme from breaking down acetylcholine, so increasing both the level and duration of action of the neurotransmitter acetylcholine. Rivastigmine is pseudoreversible inhibitor of AchE and BuChE.

Bird, T. D. "Memory loss and dementia." In Harrison's Principles of Internal.
Medicine, 15th edition, A. S. Franci, E. Daunwald, and K. J. Isrelbacher, eds.
NewYork: McGraw Hill, 2001.

4. C   Vascular dementia is the second most common form of dementia after Alzheimer's disease. In some families there is an autosomal dominant mode of inheritance, with onset around the age of 45. The term refers to a group of Syndromes caused by different mechanisms all resulting in vascular lesions in the brain. The symptoms include: (a) problems with recent memory (b) wandering or getting lost in familiar (c) places walking with rapid, shuffling steps (d) loss of bladder or bowel control(e) emotional labiality (e) difficulty following instructions and (f) problems handling money.

Tang W, Chan S, Chiu H et al (2004). Impact of applying NINDS-AIREN. criteria of probable vascular dementia to clinical and radiological characteristics of a stroke cohort with dementia". Cerebrovasc. Dis. 18 (2): 98-103.

5. B   Hachinski Ischaemic score (HIS) is based on 13 clinical features. The Hachinski ischaemic scale is an attempt to differentiate Alzheimer's type dementia and multi-infarct dementia. Other components of HIS are stepwise deterioration, fluctuating course, nocturnal confusion, relative preservation of personality, somatic complaints, emotional incontinence, associated atherosclerosis and focal neurological signs and symptoms.

Hachinski VC, Iliff LD, Zilhka E et als. (1975) Cerebral blood flow in dementia.
Arch Neurol;32:632-7.

6. C Fish consumption is considered as protective factors. Other risk factors are smoking, head injury, aluminium intake (controversial) and family history.

Lyketsos C, Colenda C, Beck C, et als (2006). Position statement of the American Association for Geriatric Psychiatry (AAGP) regarding principles of care for patients with dementia resulting from Alzheimer disease. Am J Geriatr Psychiatry 14 (7): 561-72.

7. C It is associated with late-onset Alzheimer's disease (AD).

8. D Parietal lobe damage is associated with reduced survival. Other factors are depression, prominent behavioural abnormalities, gait disturbance, congestive cardiac failure and Diabetes at base line, and more severe cognitive impairment.

J. Xie, C. Brayne, F. E Matthews, and the Medical Research Council Cognitive Function (2008). Survival times in people with dementia: analysis from population based cohort study with 14 year follow-up. BMJ, January 10, 2008 bmj.39433.616678.25v1.

9. C Short term memory and language loss are less marked in the early disease. Dementia with Lewy bodies (DLB) is one of the most common types of progressive dementia. It comprises 12-20% of dementia cases. The central feature of DLB is progressive cognitive decline, combined with three additional defining features: (1) pronounced "fluctuations" in alertness and attention, such as frequent drowsiness, lethargy, lengthy periods of time spent staring into space, or disorganized speech; (2) recurrent visual hallucinations, and (3) parkinsonian motor symptoms, such as rigidity and the loss of spontaneous movement. People may also suffer from depression.

10. A It is more common in women than men. Major depression occurs in 1-3% of the general elderly population, and an additional 8-16% have clinically significant depressive symptoms. Studies of depressed adults, indicate that those with depressive symptoms, with or without

depressive disorder, have poorer functioning, comparable to or worse than that of people with chronic medical conditions such as heart and lung disease, arthritis, hypertension, and diabetes. In addition to poor functioning, depression increases the perception of poor health, the utilization of medical services, and health care costs.

Cole G M and Dendukuri N (2003) Risk Factors for Depression Among Elderly Community Subjects: A Systematic Review and Meta-Analysis. Am J Psychiatry 160:1147-1156.

11. A   Alzheimer's disease (AD) is a neurodegenerative disease that, in its most common form, is found in people over the age of 65. Only 15% of patients suffer with thought disorder. Approximately 24million people worldwide have dementia of which the majority (~60%) is due to Alzheimer's. Clinical signs of Alzheimer's disease are characterized by progressive cognitive deterioration, together with declining activities of daily living and by neuropsychiatric symptoms or behavioural changes. It is the most common type of dementia. Plaques which contain misfolded peptides called amyloid beta (Aβ) are formed in the brain many years before the clinical signs of Alzheimer's are observed. Together, these plaques and neurofibrillary tangles form the pathological hallmarks of the disease.

Waldemar G, Dubois B, Emre M, et al (2007). "Recommendations for the diagnosis and management of Alzheimer's disease and other disorders associated with dementia: EFNS guideline". Eur. J. Neurol. 14 (1): 126.

12. B   The requirements for testamentary capacity are minimal. There are four legal criteria for determining testamentary capacity. The test generally requires that the testator is aware of:

(1)   The extent and value of their property.
(2)   The persons who are the natural beneficiaries.

(3)   The disposition they are making.

(4)   How these elements relate to form an orderly plan of distribution of property.

> Dukeminier J & Johanson S M (2005) Wills, Trusts & Estates, Sixth Edition, Aspen Publishers.

13. D   CT scan shows periventricular hypodensities and ventricular dilitation with small sulci. NPH may exhibit the classic triad of urinary incontinence, wide-based ataxic gait, and dementia (commonly referred to as "wet, wobbly and wacky"). NPH may be relieved by surgically implanting a ventriculoperitoneal shunt to drain excess cerebrospinal fluid to the abdomen where it is absorbed.

> Bateman GA, Levi CR, Schofield P, et al (2005) The pathophysiology of the aqueduct stroke volume in normal pressure hydrocephalus: can co-morbidity with other forms of dementia be excluded? Neuroradiology, 47(10): 741-8.

14. B   Levodopa responsive parkinsonism is rare. Huntington's disease (HD) is an autosomal dominant neurodegenerative disorder that displays a marked variability in its clinical manifestation and the age at which- symptoms first appear. It is characterised by hyperkinetic movements, mainly chorea, cognitive dysfunction, and psychiatric abnormalities.

> E. Gomez-Tortosa, A. et al (1998) Severity of Cognitive Impairment in Juvenile and Late-Onset Huntington Disease Arch Neurol: 55(6): 835 843.

15. B   It is fairly common to find it associated with head injury. The condition tends to occur against a background of head injury, serious illness or severe psycho-social stress. The 4 principle features are: approximate answers, clouding of consciousness, somatic conversion symptoms such as hysterical paralysis and hallucinations, visual or auditory.

> Dalfen AK, Anthony F(2000) Head injury, Dissociation and the Ganser syndrome. Brain Inj ;14(12):1101-5.

16. C Prevalence rate of OCD in old age is estimated as 0.1-0.8%.

Manela, M., Katona, C. & Livingston, G. (1996) How common are the anxiety disorders in old age? International Journal of Geriatric Psychiatry, 6: 6570.

17. D A diagnosis of AD should be considered for an individual who presents with dementia that is characterized by a gradual and progressive course of short-term memory impairment without lateralizing signs, symptoms, or lateralized cognitive deficits. Alternately, a diagnosis of VaD would be appropriate for an individual who presents with an acute onset and stepwise progression of cognitive impairment. It should be noted that the differences between AD and VaD are not always obvious. A myriad of overlapping characteristics exist between them, including the cognitive decline often associated with aging. Impairments associated with normal aging are limited to rote memory and delayed recall. In contrast, patients with AD often manifest impaired abilities to form new memories whereas patients with VaD are cognitively impaired in executive functioning activities such as organizing, planning, and initiating sequential events. The pathological hallmarks of both dementias frequently coexist, as seen in postmortem analyses of older adults with dementia. Furthermore, there is considerable overlap between risk factors associated with AD and VaD.

Levinoff JE(2007)Vascular Dementia and Alzheimer's Disease: Diagnosis and Risk Factors. Geriatrics Aging;10(1):36-41.

18. D Expressive dysphasia is a recognised feature. Frontal lobe syndrome (FLS) reflects damage to the prefrontal regions of the frontal lobe. It is characterised by deterioration in behaviour and personality in a previously normal individual. Characteristic features are (a) decreased lack of spontaneous activity (b) loss of attention - patient is disinterested and easily distracted (c) memory is normal but cannot be bothered to remember (d) loss of abstract thought (e) perseveration - tendency to continue with one form of behaviour when situation requires it to change and (f) change of affect.

Nagaratnam N, Bou-Haidar P, Leung H (2003) Confused and disturbed behaviour in the elderly following silent frontal lobe infarction.. Am J Alzheimers Dis Other Demen:18(6):333-9.

19. B   Delirium Tremens is an acute episode of delirium that is usually caused by withdrawal or abstinence from alcohol following habitual excessive drinking, or benzodiazepines or barbiturates. The mortality rate may be as high as 35% if untreated but is less than 5% with early recognition and treatment.

Wright T, Myrick H, Henderson S, Peters H, Malcolm R (2006) Risk factors for delirium tremens: a retrospective chart review. Am J Addict;15 (3):213-9.

20. C   Picks disease is a rare fronto-temporal neurodegenerative disease. It causes about 0.4-2% of all dementia and affects women more than men. The symptoms that are the most common include the decreased ability to produce language, both spoken and written aphasia, decreased planning capacity, mood swings, and personality changes.

Uchihara, T; Ikeda K, Tsuchiya K (2003) Pick body disease and Pick syndrome. Neuropathology 23 (4): 318-326.

21. D   Creutzfeldt-Jakob disease is associated with cortical dementia. Sub-cortical dementia refers to a clinical syndrome characterised by slowing of cognition, memory disturbances, difficulty with complex intellectual tasks such as strategy generation and problem solving, visuo-spatial abnormalities, and disturbances of mood and affect.

Brown, R. G. & Marsen, C. D. (1988) Sub-cortical dementia: the neuropsychological evidence. Neuroscience, 25, 363-387.

22. B   Gerstmann's syndrome is associated with parietal lesions. The inferior temporal cortex is responsible for visual perception and lesions produce inability to recognise faces, called Prosopagnosia. Lesions of the right superior temporal gyrus produce prosody.

Takeda K & Shinkeigaku R (2004),44(11):834-6.

23. B   First rank symptoms are usually present in 30%. There is strong association with deafness, although visual impairment is seen in some. Premorbid paranoid traits are present in about 45% of the patients. It is more common in females (4:1 to 9:1).

Östling & Svante (2005) Psychotic symptoms in the elderly. Current Psychosis & Therapeutics Reports 3:1.

24. C   Only 10% of cases of major depressive illness occur in old age.

25. A   Recent studies have explored a possible connection between B12 deficiency and Alzheimer's dementia but there is no clear evidence.

Morris MC, Evans DA, Schneider JA, et al (2006) Dietary folate and vitamins B-12 and B-6 not associated with incident Alzheimer's disease. J. Alzheimers Dis. 9 (4): 435-43.

26. D   Non dominant temporal lobe impairment is linked with deficits in visual memory. Autotopagnosia is agnosia that affects the sense of posture. It is characterized by an inability to localize and orient different parts of the body.

27. C   It is Receptive aphasia. This condition is suggested when the patient is unable to follow commands or questions. Speech is usually fluent but disorganized. The Wernickie's area is usually affected.

28. B   Paranoid delusions are feature of delirium tremens.

Dysmnesic syndrome is a mental disorder associated with chronic ethanol abuse (ALCOHOLISM) and nutritional deficiencies characterized by short term memory loss, confabulations, and disturbances of attention.

Adams et al.   Dysmnesic Syndrome, Alcohol-Induced. Principles of Neurology, 6th ed, p1139.

29. E   There is loss of normal fear and anger responses. Klüver-Bucy syndrome is a rare neurological disorder that causes individuals to put objects in their mouths and engage in inappropriate sexual behavior. Other symptoms may include visual agnosia, loss of normal fear and anger responses, memory loss, distractibility, seizures, and dementia. The disorder may be associated with herpes encephalitis and trauma.

Goscinski I, Kwiatkowski S, Polak J, et al.(1997) The Kluver-Bucy syndrome. J Neurosurg Sci; 41(3):269-72.

30. B   Life events commonly associated with elderly suicide are: the death of a loved one; physical illness; uncontrollable pain; fear of dying a prolonged death that damages family members emotionally and economically; social isolation and loneliness; and major changes in social roles, such as retirement. Among the elderly, white men are the most likely to die by suicide. The widowed, divorced, and recently bereaved are at high risk.

Dombrovski, Alexandre YI; Szanto, Katalin; Reynolds III, Charles F (2005) Epidemiology and risk factors for suicide in the elderly: 10-year update. Aging Health, VoL 1, No 1:135-145.

31. C   Delirium is probably the most common presenting symptom of disease in old age. Delirium, as defined in DSM-IV, is a neuropsychiatric syndrome characterized by disturbance in attention and consciousness, which develops over a short period of time and where the symptoms tend to fluctuate during the course of the day. Many studies involving elderly population with dementia and hip fracture report delirium in 20-30% preoperatively and 30-50% cases, postoperatively.

Lundström, M (2004) Delirium in old patients with femoral neck fracture: risk factors, outcome, prevention and treatment. Doctoral Thesis, Sweden.

32. C

In placebo-controlled clinical trials of elderly patients with dementia-related psychosis, the incidence of death in olanzapine-treated patients was significantly greater than placebo-treated patients (3.5% vs 1.5%, respectively). Olanzapine is not approved for the treatment of patients with dementia-related psychosis.

Schneeweiss, S (2007) Risk of death associated with the use of conventional versus atypical antipsychotic drugs among elderly patients. Canadian Medical Association Journal 176(5), pp. 627-632.

33. C

Chapter 19

Questions:
EMIs

I)   EMI Study design

A.   Cost minimisation analysis
B.   Cost effectiveness analysis
C.   Sensitivity analysis
D.   Cost benefit analysis
E.   Survival analysis
F.   Cost utility analysis

Choose the most appropriate analysis from above that should be used for each of the following scenarios.

1.   To compare the cost and consequences of two different competing interventions within a given budget for a given patient group.
2.   Analysis used to make choices between interventions for different conditions in which the units of outcome differ.
3.   If the beneficial effects of sertraline and citalopram are same in moderate depression than which drug would be more economical to use?

II)   EMI Validity

A.   Face validity
B.   Content validity
C.   Concurrent validity
D.   Construct validity

E.   Criterion validity
F.   Incremental validity
G.   Convergent validity

For each of the following statements, choose the most appropriate options from the above list.

1.   The extent to which the test measures a theoretical concept by a specific measuring device or procedure.
2.   The extent to which the test measures variables that are related to that which should be measured by the test.
3.   It demonstrates the accuracy of a measure or procedure by comparing it with another measure or procedure that has been demonstrated to be valid.

III)   EMI Substance Misuse Drug Screen

A.   1-2 days
B.   1-3 days
C.   2-4 days
D.   2-8 days
E.   7-21 days
F.   30+ days
G.   12 hours

For each of the following drugs, choose the time duration for which drug screen remains positive, from the above options.

1.   PCP
2.   Amphetamines
3.   Opiates

IV)   EMI Neurological complications of alcohol abuse

A.   Degeneration of corpus callosum
B.   Confabulation
C.   Formication

D.   Acute confusional state
E.   Opthalmoplegia
F.   Spasticity
G.   Retrograde amnesia

For each of the following condition, choose 2 most appropriate associations from the above list.

1.   Wernicke's encephalopathy
2.   Korsakoff's syndrome
3.   Marchiafava-bignami disease

V)   EMI Liaison Psychiatry, Functional symptoms

A.   Somatisation
B.   Hypochondriasis
C.   Dysmorphophobia
D.   Conversion
E.   Dissociation
F.   Functional overlay

For each of the following descriptions choose the most appropriate functional symptom from the above list.

1.   The process by which thoughts or memories unacceptable to the conscious mind are repressed from conscious expression and presents in the form of physical symptoms.
2.   Symptoms above those thought to be appropriate for the extent of organic illness.
3.   The separation of unpleasant emotions and memories from consciousness resulting in disruption of normal integrated function of consciousness.
4.   The belief that one has a particular illness despite evidence to the contrary.

VI)   EMI Liaison Psychiatry

A.   Munchausen's syndrome
B.   Dysmorphic disorder
C.   Conversion disorder
D.   Somatisation disorder
E.   Myalgic encephalomyelitis
F.   Munchausen's by proxy
G.   Somatoform pain disorder

For each of the following case scenario, choose the most appropriate diagnosis from the above options.

1.   A 21year old female who always wears loose fitting clothes to hide her figure, believing that people look at her critically due to her odd body shape. On physical examination no physical abnormality is found.

2.   30 year old male presents in the clinic with complains of lethargy, exhaustion, body aches, poor un-refreshing sleep and feels that everything has become an effort for him. During interview he is quite chatty.

3.   35 year old nurse repeatedly attends the local emergency department with her 7 years old daughter who has a wound on her arm complicated with recurrent infections.

VII)   EMI Liaison Psychiatry

A.   Wearing clothes of opposite sex for sexual pleasures.
B.   Marked unhappiness and discomfort in the birth sex.
C.   Delusional belief that a person's sex is opposite to their birth sex.
D.   Inter-sexed condition proven by karyotyping.
E.   Enduring belief that one's gender is different from their biological sex.
F.   Dressing and acting like opposite sex to work in theatres.

For the following conditions, choose 2 most appropriate associations from the above list.

1.   Transsexualism

2.   Transvestism

VIII)   EMI Defence mechanisms

A.   Denial
B.   Distortion
C.   Repression
D.   Suppression
E.   Sublimation
F.   Altruism
G.   Reaction formation

For each of the following scenarios, choose the most appropriate defence mechanism from the above options.

1.   A woman with lung cancer refuses to see a specialist but instead demands antibiotics from her GP as she believes that her difficulty in breathing is due to chest infection.
2.   A man who has racist thoughts about Afro Caribbean people start befriending black people in his neighbourhood.
3.   A man who has recently lost his house due to floods, which also killed his wife, is more concerned about his financial loss and sorting out accommodation than mourning for his dead wife and literally refuses to talk about her.

IX)   EMI Community Teams

A.   Severe and persistent mental disorder with high level of disability.
B.   Conventional community care.
C.   Short term support for non enduring mental health problems.
D.   One of the aim is to reduce the stigma associated with psychosis.
E.   Gate keeping
F.   Reducing Out-Of-Area treatments.

G.   Reduce duration of untreated psychosis (DUP).
H.   Criteria include detention under mental health act on at least one occasion in last 2 years.

For each of the following community mental health service, choose 2 most appropriate associations from the above list.

1.   Early intervention team
2.   Crisis resolution home treatment team
3.   Assertive Outreach Team

X)   EMI Drug toxicity

A.   Coarse tremors
B.   Severe muscle rigidity with bradykinesia
C.   Less severe muscle rigidity with hyperkinesias
D.   Akathesia
E.   Labile blood pressure
F.   Rapid onset and progression
G.   Slow onset and progression
H.   Tardive dyskinesia
I.   Choreoathetosis
J.   Opisthotonos

From the list above please select 3 most appropriate options for each of the following. Each option may be used once, more than once or not at all.

1.   Neuroleptic Malignant Syndrome
2.   Serotonin Syndrome
3.   Lithium toxicity

XI)   EMI Autism

A.   Angelman syndrome
B.   Down syndrome
C.   Fragile X syndrome

D.   Phenlyketonurea
E.   ADHD
F.   Pradar-Willi syndrome
G.   Rett syndrome
H.   Hurlers syndrome
I.   Hunter syndrome
J.   Tuberous sclerosis

From the list above please select one most appropriate option for each of the following. Each option may be used once, more than once or not at all.

1.   5 year old child presents with autistic symptoms, hyperphagia & hypotonia.
2.   5 year old child presents with autistic symptoms and hand wringing.
3.   5 year old child presents with autistic symptoms. His maternal grandfather & maternal uncle had the condition.

XII)   EMI - Neuropsychiatry

A.   Alcoholic hallucinosis
B.   Fahr's syndrome
C.   Alcohol withdrawal
D.   Neuroacanthosis
E.   Systemic Lupus Erythematosis
F.   Alcoholic delirium
G.   Post Herpatic encephalopathy
H.   Complex partial seizures

From the list above please select one most appropriate option for each of the following. Each option may be used once, more than once or not at all.

1.   A 40 years old homeless man is brought into A&E. He is complaining of headache, is quite agitated and confused. He had a seizure in acute medical assessment unit. MRI shows abnormal asymmetric increased signal at the right

temporal-parietal gray matter.

2. A 45 years old man recently returned from America shows aggressive behaviour. He has recently experienced seizures and has periods of fluctuating consciousness. There were tremors, muscle rigidity, a mask-like facial appearance, shuffling gait, and a "pill-rolling" motion of the fingers, on examination.

3. A 27 years old woman has sore throat, right sided facial nerve palsy and circumscribed lesions on both legs.

.————.

Chapter 20

Answers:
EMIs

I)
1.   B
2.   F
3.   A

II)
1.   D
2.   B
3.   E

III)
1.   D
2.   B
3.   A

IV)
1.   D, E
2.   B, G
3.   A, F

V)
1.   D
2.   F
3.   E
4.   B

VI)
1.   B
2.   E
3.   F

VII)
1.   B, E
2.   A, F

VIII)
1.   B
2.   G
3.   D

IX)
1.   D, G
2.   E, F
3.   A, H

X)
1.   B, E, G
2.   C, E, F
3.   A, I, J

XI)
1.   C
2.   G
3.   I

XII)
1.   G
2.   B
3.   E

Questions:
Mock Exam

You have 3 hours to complete the exam. The maximum score is 200. Each answer has one mark. Please note that each component of EMI has one mark. It is advised that the paper is attempted under exam conditions and should be completed in one sitting.
Good Luck.

1.   Commonly used statistical test for Non Parametric data include:

A.   Mean
B.   Median
C.   Standard Deviation
D.   Mode
E.   Frequencies

2.   A data is said to be continuous:

A.   If the values or observations belonging to it can be sorted according to category, for example colour
B.   If the values / observations belonging to it are distinct and separate, i.e. they can be counted (1,2,3,.....)
C.   If the values / observations belonging to it can be assigned a code in the form of a number where the numbers are simply labels. You can count but not order or measure. For example, in a data set males could be coded as 0, females as 1
D.   If the values / observations belonging to it can be ranked (put in order) or have a rating scale attached. You can count and order, but not measure. For example a rating scales of 1,2,3,4 and so on

E.   If the values / observations belonging to it may take on any value within a finite or infinite interval. You can count, order and measure data. For example height and weight

3.   The correlation coefficient between x and y is used to show:

A.   Whether y causes x
B.   Whether x is more significant than y
C.   Whether x depends upon y
D.   Whether x has any relationship with y
E.   Whether there is a linear relationship between x and y

4.   All the following studies are observational in nature except:

A.   A study of incidence of Depression in UK
B.   Comparison of 2 treatments for depression using database for the last 5 years
C.   A comparison of the outcome of patients treated with Olanzapine and Quetiapine in a RCT
D.   A study of Prevalence of schizophrenia in Germany
E.   A cohort study of people exposed to asbestos

5.   Two groups are matched for age, sex and genetic disposition. One has mental illness and the other with no mental illness. Their medical history is studied from the case notes to look for any predisposing or aetiological factors contributing to the mental illness. What kind of study is this?

A.   Randomised controlled trial
B.   Controlled trial
C.   Case control
D.   Cohort
E.   Pragmatic trial

6.   The following statement is true regarding prospective studies:

A. Existing records can be used to obtain all relevant information
B. Interviewing the carer is a necessary procedure
C. Cannot be used to study possible multiple outcomes from a single exposure
D. Are relatively less time consuming
E. They can measure the exposure without any bias in relation to the disease, as compared to retrospective studies

7. Type I error:

A. Occurs when the null hypothesis is accepted when it is in fact false
B. Occurs when the null hypothesis is accepted when it is in fact true
C. Occurs when the null hypothesis is rejected when it is in fact false
D. Occurs when the null hypothesis is rejected when it is in fact true
E. Is sometimes also referred as false negative judgement

8. A method that uses multiple variables to divide cases into meaningful and similar groups is called:

A. Multivariate ANOVA
B. Discriminant Function analysis
C. Principal components analysis
D. Canonical correlation
E. Cluster analysis

9. If John's scores in his tests were, 8,6,9,8,7,9,8 and 10. What would be the Mode in this case?

A. 6
B. 7

C.   8
D.   9
E.   10

10.   Which of the following statements about Randomised Controlled Trials is not true?

A.   Are reliable measure of efficacy
B.   Allows for meta-analysis
C.   Does not have surrogate end points
D.   Have ethical problems
E.   May suffer from volunteer bias

11.   Observational descriptive studies:

A.   Reports the differences observed between two or more groups
B.   Reports the similarities observed between two or more groups
C.   Include controlled clinical trials
D.   Are for hypothesis testing
E.   Are for hypothesis generation

12.   The following statements about 'Galbraith plot' are true except:

A.   A Galbraith plot identifies the studies which contribute most to the overall heterogeneity of the results
B.   Z statistic is on the X axis
C.   If the trials scatter about a line running through the origin at standard normal deviate zero, it suggest absence of bias
D.   Large studies tend to aggregate away from the origin
E.   The studies with heterogeneity usually lie a certain number of standard deviations above or below the line which represents the summary effect

13.   Which of the following is a parametric test?

A.   Mann Whitney U test
B.   Chi Squared test
C.   Kruskal Wallis analysis of variance
D.   Spearman rank
E.   McNemar's test

14.   Pragmatic trials:

A.   Test efficacy
B.   Blinding is easy
C.   Doesn't reflect everyday practice
D.   Test effectiveness
E.   Offer the advantage of randomisation

15.   Relative risk reduction (RRR) can be calculated by using which of the following formula?

A.   EER/CER
B.   (a/b)/(c/d)
C.   (CER-EER)/CER
D.   CER-EER
E.   1/ARR

16.   Which one of the following is not a multivariate method?

A.   Multiple regression
B.   Mann-Whitney U test
C.   Discriminant analysis
D.   Canonical correlation
E.   Factor analysis

17.   A group of people with moderate depression were chosen for a study and all were given Venlafaxine and followed up for 6 months. This is an example of:

A.   Cohort study
B.   Open trial
C.   Pragmatic trial

D.   Qualitative study
E.   Controlled trial

18.   Relative risk can be defined as:

A.   Risk of an event in one group minus the risk in the other
         group
B.   The number of patients required to be treated with the
         experimental intervention in order to prevent one
         additional adverse outcome
C.   The probability that the observed difference between the
         treatments is due to chance
D.   The ratio of odds of having the disorder in the
         experimental group relative to the odds in favour of
         having the disorder in the control group
E.   The risk of an event in one group divided by the risk in the
         other group

19.   Following are types of opiate receptors except:

A.   Alpha
B.   Kappa
C.   Lambda
D.   Delta
E.   Mu

20.   Amphetamines are associated with:

A.   Bruxism
B.   Hypotension
C.   Bradycardia
D.   Increased appetite
E.   Decreased sweating

21.   Which non-opioid medication can be used in the
         treatment of mild opioid withdrawal syndrome?

A.   Haloperidol

B.   Chlordiazepoxide
C.   Methadone
D.   Clonidine
E.   Phenytoin

22.   Which of the following is the most addictive substance of abuse?

A.   Cannabis
B.   Nicotine
C.   Cocaine
D.   Heroin
E.   PCP

23.   A drug user is brought to A&E. He has not had his usual drug for several days. He presents with tachycardia, hypertension, heperpyrexia, papillary dilatation, piloerection and rhinorrhea. What's the most likely drug responsible for his presentation?

A.   Cannabis
B.   LSD
C.   Opiates
D.   Magic mushrooms
E.   Benzodiazepines

24.   Acute harmful effects including injected conjunctivae, delayed reaction time, panic attacks, altered time sense and mild paranoia are typically associated with:

A.   Solvents
B.   Barbiturates
C.   Cannabis
D.   Cocaine
E.   Anabolic steroids

25.   Clinically significant physical dependence occurs with which of the following drugs?

A. Cocaine
B. Amphetamine
C. LSD
D. Cannabis
E. MDMA

26. Alcohol dependence syndrome described by Edwards and Gross constitute the following features except

A. Primacy of alcohol seeking behaviour
B. Narrowing of repertoire
C. Craving
D. Loss of control of consumption
E. Continued use despite negative consequences

27. Which of the following is a risk factor for Alcoholism?

A. Family history of Schizophrenia
B. Non alcoholic biological father but alcoholism in adoptive father
C. Male sex
D. Family history of Anxiety
E. Young female

28. In terms of Alcohol use, which one of the following statement is not true?

A. In the UK roughly 93% of men drink alcohol
B. In the UK roughly 87% of the women drink alcohol
C. The distinction between normal and heavy drinker is arbitrary
D. Greater number of alcohol-related problems occur in normal rather than heavy drinkers
E. The term 'Alcoholic' is used in DSM-IV but not in ICD-10

29. Which of the following test is more specific for alcohol related liver damage?

A.   Gamma GT
B.   CK
C.   MCV
D.   CDT
E.   MCHC

30.   Which of the following statements about Acamprosite is
        true?

A.   It is also called Antabuse
B.   It blocks the aldehyde dehydrogenise enzyme
C.   It causes extremely unpleasant side effects when used
        with alcohol
D.   It reduces craving for alcohol
E.   It works by behaving as negative reinforcer

31.   Amphetamines mainly act by:

A.   Inhibiting the reuptake of neurotransmitters
B.   Releasing stored monoamines in the synaptic cleft
C.   Increasing affinity of GABA a receptors
D.   Blocking dopamine receptors
E.   Blocking nor epinephrine receptors

32.   The lifetime prevalence of nicotine dependence in the
        general population is:

A.   5%
B.   10%
C.   15%
D.   20%
E.   25%

33.   What's the peak time for withdrawal syndrome after the
        cessation of heroin use?

A.   12 Hours

B.   48 hours
C.   72 hours
D.   5 days
E.   1 week

34.   A 40 year old male who has gained good insight into his problems after 6 months of Psychodynamic Therapy starts turning up late at sessions and regularly insists on cancelling his appointments. Which of the following process is most relevant?

A.   Acting out
B.   Resistance
C.   Abreaction
D.   Projection
E.   Manipulation

35.   The principles on which long term supportive psychotherapy is based, best apply to:

A.   Patients with history of remission
B.   Patients with first episode psychosis
C.   Patients with complex illness and treatment resistant psychosis
D.   Patients with functional illness as well as personality disorder
E.   Patients with early onset psychosis

36.   The feelings and patterns of behaviour in the patient, towards the therapist, which unconsciously partly represents their earlier relationships in life, is called:

A.   Splitting
B.   Projection
C.   Identification
D.   Isolation
E.   Transference

37.   A woman who has been a victim of domestic violence, says
       that it was probably a good thing that she was abused
       because she has learnt a lot from life and would be more
       careful in future relationships. Which of the following ego
       defence mechanism is likely to be involved here?

A.   Denial
B.   Distortion
C.   Turning against the self
D.   Reaction formation
E.   Intellectualisation

38.   Negative Therapeutic Reaction:

A.   Usually occurs when patient does not like the therapist
B.   Usually occurs when therapist does not like the patient
C.   When both patient and therapist don't get on
D.   Is a sign of hidden feelings of guilt and shame
E.   Is the first sign of transference

39.   In Group Therapy:

A.   One important aim is to abolish the hierarchy
B.   Once decided leaders cannot be changed
C.   Altruism is a common therapeutic factor
D.   In the absence of an autocratic leader the groups runs
      smoothly
E.   The therapist encourage pairing

40.   EMDR is taught in:

A.   6 stages
B.   8 stages
C.   10 stages
D.   12 stages
E.   16 stages

41.   Automatic thoughts are one type of cognitive errors

identified in CBT. Which one of the following is not an automatic thought?

A. Selective abstraction
B. All or nothing thinking
C. Catastrophic thinking
D. Over generalisation
E. Displacement

42. 'Reality based' short-term therapy aimed at 'cognitive restructuring' developed by Albert Ellis in 1995 is called:

A. Cognitive Analytic Therapy
B. Rational Emotive Therapy
C. Behavioural therapy
D. Dialectical behaviour Therapy
E. Cognitive Behaviour Therapy

43. 'Goodbye letters' are written in:

A. Cognitive Analytic Therapy
B. Dialectical behaviour Therapy
C. Rational Emotive Therapy
D. Interpersonal Therapy
E. Cognitive Behaviour Therapy

44. All of the following diseases have been associated with Apolipoprotein E gene (APOE) except:

A. Late-onset Alzheimer's disease (AD)
B. Hyperlipoproteinemia type III
C. Diabetes mellitus
D. Atherosclerosis
E. Non Diabetic Nephropathy

45. EEG in patients with Alzheimer's disease (AD) is not associated with:

A.   Increased beta activity
B.   Slowing in alpha waves
C.   Increased theta waves
D.   Increased delta
E.   EEG data helps distinguish a potential Alzheimer's patient from a severely depressed person, whose brain waves are normal

46. Which statement is not true about Persecutory delusions in elderly?

A.   10-15% of elderly patients suffer with persecutory delusions
B.   Schneider's first rank symptoms may be associated
C.   They respond well to anti-psychotic treatment
D.   Persecutory delusions may precede the onset of dementia
E.   Persecutory delusions are usually shared by their partners

47. A 67 years old man was referred to outpatient with memory problem for past 12 months. His wife was concerned that short term memory has deteriorated recently but long term memory is better preserved. The most appropriate next step would be:

A.   Full history, physical and neurological examination
B.   MSE, including full cognitive assessment
C.   CT scan of head
D.   All of the above
E.   None of the above

48. General principles of prescribing in old age include all of the following except:

A.   Start at a very low dose
B.   The elderly are particularly prone to EPSEs
C.   Typical neuroleptics are better tolerated than atypical
D.   Beware of drug interactions due to common problem of polypharmacy

E.   Maximum efficacy is often achieved with low doses

49.   All of the following is associated with Pseudodementia
          except:

A.   The episode tends to start with depressive symptoms
B.   Patient often complains of memory problem and wants
          help
C.   It is an ICD-10 diagnosis
D.   Rapid onset
E.   Apraxia and aphasia is usually absent

50.   Late onset schizophrenia differs from young onset
          schizophrenia by:

A.   Persecutory delusions often predominate
B.   First rank symptoms are more common
C.   Cognitive symptoms are very mild
D.   Partition delusions are common
E.   Presence of sensory impairment

51.   All of the following are true regarding Lewy bodies (LB)
          except:

A.   The lewy bodies are insoluble complexes formed within
          neurons by phosphorylation of neurofilament proteins by
          proteins kinases
B.   LB occur in Parkinson's disease
C.   LB occur in normal aging
D.   Primary autonomic failure is associated with LB
E.   Commonly seen in dementia of lewy body type (DLB)

52.   Recognised features of Alzheimer's disease include all of
          the following except:

A.   Mirror sign
B.   Finger agnosia
C.   Logoclonia

D. Rarely associated epilepsy
E. Visual agnosia

53. All of the following features are more likely in delirium than in dementia except:

A. Lability of affect
B. Visual hallucinations
C. Insidious onset
D. Perceptual abnormality
E. Restlessness

54. Which one of the following features is predictor of poor outcome in conduct disorder?

A. Female gender
B. Family criminality
C. High IQ
D. Competence at a skill
E. Warm relationship with a key adult

55. Which one of the following disorders is not included as Pervasive Developmental Disorder in DSM-IV?

A. Autism
B. Asperger's syndrome
C. Childhood schizophrenia
D. Childhood disintegrative disorder
E. Rett's syndrome

56. Which of following statements is not correct regarding Juvenile Delinquency?

A. More common in males
B. A juvenile delinquent is a person who has not yet reached the age of majority
C. It is a legal term and not a psychiatric diagnosis
D. Anti social behaviour may be normal part of growing up

E.   Many will meet criteria for conduct disorder

57.   Increased risk factors for child sexual abuse include all of
         the following except:
A.   Gay, lesbian and bisexual youth
B.   Mental illness
C.   Physical/mental disability
D.   Conflict with or between parents
E.   Too many friends

58.   Recognised features of Emotional Disorders in children
         and adolescents include all of the following except:

A.   Sleep and cortisol studies show no abnormalities unlike
         adults
B.   Phobias are emotional disorders
C.   Suicide methods are simple
D.   More common in females before puberty
E.   Sleep and appetite is less affected than adults

59.   Factors that predispose to persistent nocturnal enuresis
         include all of the following except:

A.   It is more likely to be persistent bed wetting in children
         with delayed developmental milestones
B.   Down's syndrome is a risk factor
C.   Mother aged less than 20 at time of birth
D.   Early potty training prevents bedwetting
E.   Airways obstruction with snoring increases risk

60.   Separation anxiety disorder of childhood is associated
         with all of the following except:

A.   There should be no generalized disturbance of personality
         development of functioning
B.   It excludes neurotic disorders
C.   ICD-10 code F53.0 is applicable
D.   Persistent reluctance or refusal to go to school because of

fear of separation

E. It runs in the families

61. Childhood stuttering presents with all of the following features except:

A. Strong association with major mental illness
B. More common in boys
C. Significant family history
D. 40% of children will outgrow the problem
E. No known genetic factors at present

62. Recognised features of Encoprosis include all of the following except:

A. Associated with constipation
B. Occurs equally in boys and girls
C. It is faecal soiling with the loss of semi-formed or usually liquid stools
D. Usually associated with meningomyelocele
E. Children are often referred to CAMHS

63. All of the following features are associated with Narcolepsy except:

A. Cataplexy
B. Occurs equally in males and females
C. Hypnogogic hallucinations
D. Sleep paralysis
E. Rapid eye movement sleep disorder

64. Which one of the following is unlikely to be associated with depression in children?

A. Irritable mood
B. Mood congruent auditory hallucinations
C. Pervasive anhedonia
D. Suicidal ideation
E. Occurs commonly in school age boys

65.   A medical registrar asks you to see a patient with
        Parkinson's disease, presenting with mania like
        symptoms. Which of the following statements regarding
        Parkinson's disease is false?

A.   High comorbidity with affective disorders
B.   The close relatives of people with Parkinson's disease are
        at increased risk for depression and anxiety
C.   High risk of psychiatric disorders
D.   The average age of onset is 45 years
E.   Parkinsonian symptoms rarely may appear in people
        before the age of 20.

66.   All of the following genes have been associated with
        Parkinson's disease except:

A.   Parkin
B.   DJ-3
C.   PINK1
D.   LRRK2
E.   Alpha-synuclein

67.   Olfactory hallucinations are commonly seen in which one
        of the following conditions?

A.   Schizophrenia
B.   Partial complex seizures
C.   Wilson disease
D.   Somotisation disorder
E.   Hypochondriasis

68.   All of the following statements regarding chronic
        medically unexplained fatigue are correct except:

A.   Classified as Neurasthenia in ICD-10
B.   Sometimes referred as Fibromylgia
C.   Associated with Chronic Lyme disease
D.   Comes under Undifferentiated somatisation disorders in

DSM-IV

E.   Usually there is no history of previous depressive episodes

69.   Vulnerable groups to develop Hypochondriasis includes the following:

A.   Muslim people
B.   Men
C.   Plumbers
D.   Young people
E.   Higher social class

70.   Addison's disease can present with all of the following psychiatric features except:

A.   Excessive energy
B.   Fatigue
C.   Low mood
D.   Anxiety
E.   Apathy

71.   All of the following statements regarding chronic fatigue syndrome (CFS) are correct except:

A.   There are no diagnostic tests
B.   Herpes virus is commonly associated
C.   Hypocortisolism is associated with one third of the cases
D.   Multijoint pain without swelling or redness
E.   Impairment in short-term memory and concentration

72.   A midwife asked you for a home visit, to see a 24 years old woman, who gave birth to her first child nearly two weeks ago. She is acting bizarrely and appears to be responding to unseen external stimuli. You suspect puerperal psychosis. What would be the most appropriate action at this stage?

A.   Full Psychiatric assessment
B.   To consider child's safety
C.   Admission in mother and baby unit if available
D.   All of the above
E.   None of the above

73.   All of the following statements are true regarding transsexualism except:

A.   Prevalence of 1 in 30 000 for female to male transsexuals
B.   Transvestism is not same as transsexualism
C.   Inter sexed condition can be ruled out by normal karyotyping
D.   Schizophrenia is included in differential diagnosis
E.   Genital mutilation is rare

74.   Which one of the following is not recognised in Body Dysmorphic disorder (BDD)?

A.   It may be a delusional disorder
B.   Higher preoccupations with genitals and excessive body hair among male patients
C.   Mostly present to psychiatrists first
D.   SSRIs are useful drugs for pharmacological treatment
E.   NICE guidelines do not recommend use of tricyclic antidepressants

75.   Which of the following is associated with delinquency?

A.   Number of children in school
B.   High pupil to teacher ratio
C.   More academic emphasis in school
D.   Frequency and quality of school outings
E.   High punishment and low praise

76.   Sex Offender Treatment Programme (SOTP) used in prisons and hospitals for sex offenders can be described as:

A.   Cognitive analytic therapy
B.   Group behaviour therapy
C.   Psychodynamic therapy
D.   Group cognitive behaviour therapy
E.   Schematherapy

77.   HCR-20:

A.   Can be expected to yield accurate outcomes with all types of patients and under all manner of conditions
B.   Is the last step in the risk assessment process
C.   Is a substitute for basic good sense and judgement
D.   Makes the basis for decision making more transparent
E.   Should be used only in research settings

78.   When considering discharging a patient from a secure hospital, which of the following should be part of your Care Programme Approach?

A.   Assessment of need and risk
B.   Agreeing a package of care with your patient
C.   Nominating a key worker
D.   Regular review and monitoring of the care plan
E.   All of the above

79.   Responsivity principle in offender treatment refers to:

A.   Whether or not the person is responsive to treatment
B.   Treatability of the patient
C.   Barriers to the patients treatment
D.   Adapting the treatment for the particular characteristics and abilities of the patient group being treated
E.   Patients response to similar treatments in the past

80.   Which of the following is a crucial item in the assessment of dangerousness?

A.   Details of index event and its antecedents

B.   History of substance misuse
C.   Psychosexual behaviour and interests
D.   Attitude to treatment
E.   All of the above

81.   The commonest mode of death in prison is:

A.   Hanging
B.   Cardiovascular death
C.   HIV related
D.   Self poisoning
E.   Starvation

82.   Which is the most common disorder among the mentally
         disordered offenders who commit homicide?

A.   Alcohol and drug dependence
B.   Personality disorder
C.   Schizophrenia
D.   Delusional disorder
E.   Depression

83.   Among the prison population which one of the following
         is the commonest psychiatric disorder?

A.   Schizophrenia
B.   Depression
C.   Mania/hypomania
D.   Anxiety
E.   Personality disorder and substance misuse

84.   With regards to incest which of the following statement is
         not correct?

A.   It is a synonym of paedophilia
B.   Sexual relationship between step father and step daughter
         is not considered to be incest
C.   If the female is above 16 years of age and consents to sex

knowingly that the person is her brother or father does not amount to incest

D.   In mother-son incest mother usually has a neurotic disorder

E.   In father-daughter incest father rarely has psychiatric disorder

85.   At 3%, the point prevalence of Schizophrenia in populations considered to have mild idiopathic intellectual disability is some:

A.   Two times that in the general population
B.   Three times that is the general population
C.   Four times that is the general population
D.   Five times that is the general population
E.   Same as that is the general population

86.   For the purposes of defining learning disability, the condition manifests before the age of:

A.   21 years
B.   18 years
C.   16 years
D.   13 years
E.   10 years

87.   For diagnosing epilepsy which of the following investigation is best used to detect areas of hypometabolism in brain?

A.   CT scan
B.   MRI scan
C.   EEG
D.   Video EEG
E.   SPECT

88.   In the patient group with Down's syndrome who are over 40 yrs of age and also have Alzhiemer's Dementia and

epilepsy, the seizures are usually:

A. Febrile convulsions
B. Tonic clonic
C. Myoclonic
D. Absence seizures
E. Atonic seizures

89. The first line drug of treatment in adults with LD having myoclonic seizure is:

A. Lamotrigine
B. Sodium Valproate
C. Carbamazepine
D. Levetiracetam
E. Topiramate

90. Which one of the following is not an Autosomal dominant condition?

A. α- Thalassaemia mantal retardation
B. Neurofibromatosis
C. Tuberous sclerosis
D. Sturge-weber syndrome
E. Von Hippel-Lindau syndrome

91. What percentage of patients with Tuberous Sclerosis, suffer with seizures?

A. 10%
B. 30%
C. 50%
D. 70%
E. 90%

92. All of the following are X-linked recessive conditions except:

A.   Hunter Syndrome
B.   Fragile X syndrome
C.   Lesch-Nyhan syndrome
D.   Oculocerebrorenal syndrome of Lowe
E.   Fabry disease

93.   What percentage of mild LD cases are caused by maternal alcohol use?

A.   10-20%
B.   30-40%
C.   50-60%
D.   70%
E.   80%

94.   Pseudo-mature language ability in some, that are initially affectionate and engaging, and later become anxious, hyperactive and uncooperative, represents a behaviour phenotype for:

A.   Williams Syndrome
B.   Smith-Magenis Syndrome
C.   Prader-Willi Syndrome
D.   Fragile X Syndrome
E.   Down's Syndrome

95.   In which of the following patients you will not consider CT head?

A.   First episode of psychosis
B.   Movement disorder in antipsychotic naive patient
C.   First episode of depression
D.   Personality change
E.   Memory loss

96.   Poor prognostic factors in schizophrenia, does not include which of the following?

A.   Insidious onset
B.   Onset in childhood/adolescence
C.   Cognitive impairment
D.   Poor pre-morbid adjustment
E.   Marked mood disturbance

97.   Which of the following is a characteristic finding on brain
        CT/MRI scans in schizophrenia?

A.   Enlarged ventricles
B.   Reduction in brain volume
C.   Enlarged cortical sulci
D.   Cerebellar atrophy
E.   None of the above

98.   Which of the following is not a good prognostic factor in
        depression?

A.   Acute onset
B.   Endogenous depression
C.   Earlier age of onset
D.   Neuroticism
E.   Good social support

99.   A 32 year old man with first episode of depression has
        been successfully treated with citalopram 40mg daily. He
        does not have any residual symptoms. Which of the
        following is correct?

A.   Continue with same dose indefinitely
B.   Reduce dose to 20 mg and continue indefinitely
C.   Continue for another 2 years and then gradually reduce
        and discontinue
D.   Continue for another 6 months and then gradually reduce
        and discontinue
E.   Reduce to 20 mg and stop over next 6 weeks

100.   Which of the following is correct regarding, Physical

illness which can mimic a manic / hypomanic presentation?

A.   Cushing's syndrome
B.   HIV
C.   Brain tumour
D.   SLE
E.   All of the above

101.   A 35 year old female with bipolar affective disorder current episode depression is currently on fluoxetine 40 mg and lithium 800mg daily. She presents with coarse tremors, ataxia, slurring of speech and excitement. Which of the following is most likely?

A.   Mania
B.   Serotonin syndrome
C.   Neuroleptic malignant syndrome
D.   Lithium toxicity
E.   None of the above

102.   Which of the following is a symptom of pathological grief?

A.   Excessive guilt
B.   Hallucinations in addition to the images and voices of the deceased
C.   Prolonged period of not being able to function normally
D.   Thoughts of death
E.   All of the above

103.   Up to what percentage of patients with schizophrenia have OCD?

A.   20%
B.   30%
C.   40%
D.   50%
E.   60%

104.   Which of the following is the most consistent finding on
        neuro-imaging in PTSD?

A.   Enlarged ventricles
B.   Hippocampus volume reduction
C.   Caudate volume reduction
D.   Abnormality of prefrontal cortex
E.   All of the above

105.   In severe OCD several PET studies have shown
        abnormalities in:

A.   Caudate nuclei
B.   Hypothalamus
C.   Hippocampus
D.   Temporal lobe
E.   Thalamus

106.   What is the rate of depression in OCD?

A.   10%
B.   30%
C.   50%
D.   70%
E.   None of the above

107.   Which of the following disorders has the highest mortality
        rate among all the psychiatric disorders?

A.   Schizophrenia
B.   Depression
C.   Bipolar affective disorder
D.   Anorexia nervosa
E.   Personality disorder

108.   Which of the following has best evidence in treatment for
        bulimia nervosa?

A.   CBT
B.   IPT
C.   Psychodynamic psychotherapy
D.   CAT
E.   Self help manuals

109.   Which of the following is true for thyroid function test in anorexia nervosa?

A.   Low thyroxine with increased TSH
B.   High thyroxine with low TSH
C.   High thyroxine with high TSH
D.   Low thyroxine with normal TSH
E.   Low thyroxine with low TSH

110.   Which of the following medications increase sex drive?

A.   Mirtazapine
B.   Venlafaxine
C.   Clomipramine
D.   Imipramine
E.   Sertraline

111.   With regards to the role of hospital admission in management of personality disorder which of the following statement is true?

A.   They benefit from prolonged admissions
B.   In presentations with axis I disorder admission is not beneficial
C.   Long term admission should be to therapeutic community
D.   Crisis admission usually requires long term stay
E.   All of the above

112.   With regards to progression of personality disorders which of the following is true?

A.   Cluster A patients generally improve with age

B.   Cluster B patients generally remain unchanged with age
C.   Cluster C patients generally worsen with age
D.   20% of schizotypal personality disorder patients develop schizophrenia
E.   When patients with obsessional personality disorder worsen with age they are more likely to develop depression than OCD

113.   Following an acute episode of schizophrenia which of the following is common?

A.   Social phobia
B.   Generalised anxiety disorder
C.   Post psychotic depression
D.   PTSD
E.   Panic disorder

114.   Evaluation of social care needs in chronic mentally ill patients is used for:

A.   Tracking individual recovery
B.   Monitoring residual symptoms
C.   Cost effectiveness
D.   Ascertain professional's view
E.   All of the above

115.   All of the following are characteristics of an individual vulnerable to developing PTSD except

A.   Repressive coping style
B.   Female gender
C.   Past psychiatric history
D.   Previous traumatisation and peri-traumatic dissociative experiences
E.   Denial of trauma

116.   A 38 year old man with recurrent depressive disorder has been successfully treated with mirtazapine 45mg daily. He

does not have any residual symptoms. His previous depressive episode was 2 years ago. Which of the following applies?

A.   Continue treatment for at least 5 years
B.   Continue treatment for at least 4 years
C.   Continue treatment for at least 3 years
D.   Continue treatment for at least 2 years
E.   Continue treatment for at least 1 year

117. Which of the following medication should be stopped before giving ECT?
A.   Lithium
B.   Olanzapine
C.   Sertraline
D.   Venlafaxine
E.   All of the above

118. Which of the following is true for prognosis of schizoaffective disorder?

A.   Better than that for mood disorder
B.   Worse than that for schizophrenia
C.   Better than that for schizophrenia
D.   Same as that for schizophrenia
E.   Same as that for mood disorder

119. Which of the following is not a good prognostic factor for bipolar affective disorder?

A.   Male sex
B.   Later age of onset
C.   Brief manic episodes
D.   Few comorbid physical health problems
E.   Few psychotic symptoms

120. For refractory bipolar depression which of the following should be used?

A.   Lithium
B.   Lamotrigine
C.   Carbamazepine
D.   Risperidone
E.   Topiramate

121.   Which of the following medication may produce anxiety like symptoms?

A.   Antihypertensives
B.   Bronchodilators
C.   Anticholinergics
D.   Disulfiram
E.   All of the above

122.   What is the most common cause of death in anorexia nervosa?

A.   Suicide
B.   Cardiac complications
C.   Renal failure
D.   Accidents
E.   Infection leading to sepsis

123.   Which of the following is not a poor prognostic factor for anorexia nervosa?

A.   Male sex
B.   Early onset
C.   Chronic illness
D.   Bulimic symptoms
E.   Poor parental relationship

124.   Which of the following hampers the good prognosis in bulimia nervosa?

A.   Anxiety
B.   Severe personality disorder

C.   OCD
D.   Schizophrenia
E.   None of the above

125.   Which of the following is the most common cause of hypersomnia?

A.   Narcolepsy
B.   Kleine-Levin syndrome
C.   Idiopathic hypersomnia
D.   Insufficient sleep syndrome
E.   Post traumatic hypersomnia

126.   With regards to psychopharmacological therapy in personality disorder which of the following is true?

A.   Antipsychotics have shown some benefits for cluster A and cluster B disorders
B.   Lithium and anticonvulsants have shown some benefits with impulsivity and affective instability
C.   Antidepressants have shown some benefits in borderline and cluster C disorders
D.   The main indication is for comorbid axis I disorders
E.   All of the above

127.   In patients with chronic schizophrenia on long term antipsychotics which of the following scale is useful to objectively monitor for any abnormal involuntary movements?

A.   Lunzer's scale
B.   AIMS
C.   BDI
D.   HDRS
E.   All of the above

128.   In patients with schizophrenia which of the following is true?

A.   Family therapy reduces relapse
B.   No evidence for CBT in relapse prevention
C.   No evidence for compliance therapy in relapse prevention
D.   Depot medication does not reduce relapse rate
E.   All of the above

129.   All of the following can reduce libido except

A.   Depression
B.   Injury to spinal cord
C.   Multiple sclerosis
D.   Increased prolactin levels
E.   Chronic pain

130.   Which of the following is a co-morbid disorder with
           trichotillomania?

A.   OCD
B.   Personality disorder
C.   Generalised anxiety disorder
D.   Depression
E.   All of the above

EMIs

I.   EMI - Study design Strengths

A.   Quick to perform
B.   Good for studying rare exposures
C.   Cheaper than RCT
D.   Eliminates all biases
E.   Perfect matching (patients as their own controls)
F.   Useful for studying aetiology
G.   Can study the treatment of rare disease.
H.   Can assess multiple outcomes

         For each of the study design below, choose 3 strengths
         from the above options. Any option can be used more than

once.

131-133. Case control study

134-136. Crossover trial

137-139. Cohort study

II.   EMI - Study design Flaws

A.   Selection bias
B.   Observation bias
C.   Confounding
D.   Publication bias
E.   Allocation bias
F.   Little statistical power
G.   Drowning of important effects

For each of the following study below, choose 3 most likely flaws from the above options. Any option can be used more than once

140-142. A study comparing 2 different treatments for depression involving patients from a small practice divided into 2 groups by the clinicians. The patients are matched for age, sex and co morbid conditions. The patients are not aware of the treatment they are receiving.

143-145. Systematic review of RCTs, studying treatments for Bipolar affective disorder. Researchers selected RCTs by searching the internet medical databases for all the published studies. Independent reviewers compiled the results of all findings with the help of meta analysis.

III.   EMI - Statistical tests

A.   Unpaired t test
B.   Paired t test

C.   Wilcoxon matched pairs test
D.   One way analysis of variance
E.   Kruskal Wallis analysis of variance
F.   Chi squared test
G.   McNemar's test
H.   Regression
I.   Multiple regression

Choose the most appropriate test from above for each of the following statements.

146.   Non parametric test to assess 3 or more sets of observations from same sample

147.   Parametric test assessing numerical relationship between 2 quantitative variables, allowing one value to be predicted from another

148.   Non parametric test used to assess whether the chances of getting into a grammar school increases if you are from a higher social class

149.   Parametric test allowing you to compare 2 diagnostic tests applied to the same sample

IV.   EMI - Psychological therapies

A.   Paraprexes
B.   Free ranging discussion
C.   Free association
D.   Amplification
E.   Psychotherapy file
F.   Role transitions
G.   Validation
H.   3Rs (Recognition, Reformulation and Revision)

For each of the following type of Therapies, choose 2 most appropriate associations from the above options.

150-151. Dynamic Therapy

152-153. Group Therapy

154-155. Cognitive Analytic Therapy

V.   EMI Causes of learning disability

A.   Down's syndrome
B.   Fragile X syndrome
C.   Tuberous sclerosis
D.   Klienfelter syndrome
E.   Foetal alcohol syndrome
F.   Rett syndrome
G.   Phenylketonuria
H.   Angelman syndrome
I.   Smith-Magenis syndrome
J.   Turner's syndrome

From the list above please select one most appropriate answer for the following statements. Each option may be used once, more than once or not at all.

156.   It is the commonest known cause of learning disability in western countries

157.   It is a disorder of unknown aetiology, may be associated with MECP2 gene at Xq28, and   exclusively affects girls

158.   It is a preventable cause of severe learning disability

159.   It is a commonest inherited cause of learning disability

160.   It is a commonest genetic cause of learning disability

161.   It is an autosomal recessive condition

162.   It is an autosomal dominant condition

163. It is an X-linked dominant condition

VI. EMI Clinical features of syndromes associated with LD

A. Self hugging
B. Brushfield's spot
C. Hyperphagia
D. Severe sleep problems
E. Single palmar crease
F. Hand flapping
G. Salaam attacks
H. Hypogenitalism
I. Ash leaf spots
J. Large testicles

From the list above please select the two most relevant clinical features for the following syndromes. Each option may be used once, more than once or not at all.

164-165. Prader-Willi syndrome

166-167. Down's syndrome

168-169. Smith-Magenis syndrome

170-171. Fragile X syndrome

172-173. Tuberous sclerosis

VII. EMI Co-morbidity between personality disorders and other mental disorders

A. Paranoid personality disorder
B. Schizoid personality disorder
C. Schizotypal personality disorder
D. Antisocial personality disorder
E. Borderline personality disorder
F. Narcissistic personality disorder
G. Histrionic personality disorder

H.   Avoidant personality disorder
I.   Dependent personality disorder
J.   Obsessive compulsive personality disorder

From the list above please select the type of personality disorder which has the strongest association with the following mental illnesses. Each option may be used once, more than once or not at all.

174.   Bulimia nervosa

175.   Social phobia

176.   Schizophrenia

177.   Substance misuse

178.   Delusional disorder

179.   Post traumatic stress disorder

VIII.   EMI Level of security

A.   Admit to open ward
B.   Admit to PICU / low secure unit
C.   Admit to medium secure unit
D.   Admit to personality disorder unit at high secure hospital
E.   Admit to DSPD unit
F.   Transfer to open ward
G.   Transfer to PICU / low secure unit
H.   Transfer to medium secure unit
I.   Transfer to high secure unit
J.   Transfer to DSPD unit
K.   To remain in the current institution

From the above list select the most appropriate option for the following scenarios. Each option may be used once, more than once or not at all.

180.   A 24-year-old man with a significant forensic history including four counts of grievous bodily harm and threats to kill was assessed by forensic psychiatrist at the end of his current sentence for threats to kill. The assessment concluded that his PCL-R score was 23 and he had definite DSM IV diagnosis of borderline personality disorder and antisocial personality disorder, and he posed a grave and immediate danger to the public.

181.   A 31 year old man with chronic schizophrenia who was transferred to medium secure unit from high secure unit 2 months ago where he had spent 2 years after killing his girlfriend. He took one of the patients as hostage and demanded to be discharged. Situation was diffused and he apologised afterwards.

182.   A 25 year old male patient with bipolar affective disorder presents with a manic episode. He has history of criminal damage and assaulting a staff member during his recent admission, 2 months ago when he had similar symptoms.

183.   A 32 year old male with a diagnosis of schizophrenia and an index offence of homicide has been at the high secure hospital for 7 years. He has been symptom free for 3 years and has engaged in psychological work related to index offence. There have not been any untoward incidents to report in the last 2 years. He however has history of abrupt relapses getting unwell within days.

IX.   EMI - Substance misuse

A.   Flashbacks
B.   Local anaesthetic effect
C.   Bruxism
D.   TLE
E.   Conjunctival injection
F.   Brain atrophy
G.   Reduces intraocular pressure in Glaucoma

H.   Formication
I.   Hypertension
J.   Lacrimation

For each of the following substances choose most appropriate associations from the above list.

184-185. Marijuana (two answers)

186-187. Copper (inhalant) (two answers)

188-189. Cocaine- (two answers)

190.   PCP (one answer)

X.   EMI - Features of Dementia

A.   Intra cytoplasmic neuronal inclusions.
B.   Severe knife edge atrophy of the frontal and temporal lobe.
C.   Neurofibrillary tangles.
D.   Periventricular hypodensities on CT scan.
E.   Multi-infarcts.
F.   Stepwise progression.

Select one feature from the above list, for each of the following conditions:

191.   Pick's disease

192.   Normal pressure hydrocephalus

193.   Dementia of lewy body type

194.   Alzheimer's disease

XI.   EMI - Anti-dementia Drugs

A.   Memantine

B.   Donepezil
C.   Rivastigmine
D.   Galantamine
E.   Naltrexone Hydrochloride
F.   Aripiprazole

Please choose one option from the above list, that best fits
with the statements below:

195.   Long half life, once daily dose, less adverse effects, max.
         dose 10 mg daily.

196.   No potential for interaction, can be used in Parkinson's
         diseases, max dose 6 mg x b.d.

197.   Moderate to severe dementia, rare association with
         suicidal ideation, max. dose 10 mg x b.d.

XII.   EMI - Pharmacological Treatment of ADHD

A.   Methylphenidate
B.   Clonidine
C.   Risperidone
D.   Atomoxetine
E.   Dexamphetamine
F.   Modafinal

Please choose one option from the above list that best fits
with the statements below:

198.   Generally well tolerated, recommended by NICE,
         worsening of tics, max. dose 60 mg / day.

199.   Not a controlled drug, NA reuptake inhibitor, less
         problem with sleep and appetite.

200.   Useful in the presence of tics, regular monitoring of BP,
         off license use.

. ———— .

Answers:
Mock Exam

1. B   Non-Parametric statistics do not rely upon normally distributed continuous data with equal variances.

Wasserman L 2007, All of Non Parametric statistics, Springer.

2. E   A is the definition of categorical data. B is the definition of discrete data. C is the definition of Nominal data. D is the definition of Ordinal data. E is the definition of Continuous data.

Statistics Glossary v1.1, Valerie J. Easton and John H. McColl.

3. E

4. C   Experimental

5. C

6. E   For example cohort studies.

7. D

8. B

9. C   Mode is the number that occurs most frequently. (6,7,8,8,8,9,10)

10. C

11. E

12. B   Galbraith plot is used to identify the studies which contribute most to the overall heterogeneity of the results. Z statistic is on the Y axis and 1/SE on the X axis.

13. E

14. D   Pragmatic trials include all patients with a particular disorder in a given location and therefore have generalisability.

15. C

16. B

17. B

18. E

19. A

20. A

21. D

22. B

23. C   Withdrawal symptoms

24. C

25. A

26. C   Craving is part of CAGE, a 4-item questionnaire used as a screen for alcohol problems.

27. C

28. E

29. D

30. D

31. B

32. D

33. B

34. B

35. C

36. E

37. E

38. D (Sigmund Freud papers, The Ego and the Id)

39. C

40. B

41. E

42. B

43. A

44. E Diabetes mellitus type-1 and 2 both have association with Apolipoprotein E gene (APOE) but there is no conclusive evidence to support link with non-Diabetic nephropathy.

G. Liew, A. Shankar, J. J. Wang et al (2007) Apolipoprotein E Gene Polymorphisms and Retinal Vascular Signs: The Atherosclerosis Risk in Communities (ARIC) Study Arch Ophthalmol; 125(6): 813 818.

45. A   There is slowing of beta activity.

46. E

47. D

48. C   Start at low dose and increase slowly. Dangerous side effects may happen even with low doses. Suicide risk needs to be considered, as old age is a risk factor for suicide.

Spinewine, K. Schmader, N. Barber et al. Appropriate prescribing in elderly people: how well can it be measured and optimised? The Lancet, Volume 370, Issue 9582, Pages 173-184.

49. C   Pseudodementia is a state of general apathy resembling dementia, but due to a psychiatric disorder rather than organic brain disease and potentially reversible.

50. B   First rank symptoms are less common. Partition delusion is a firmly held belief that a person or object can pass through a barrier.

51. C   Lewy bodies do not occur in normal aging.

Mckeith (1994) BJPsych:165; 324-32.

52. D   Epilepsy is fairly common. Logoclonia is spasmodic repetition of words or parts of words, particularly the end syllables, often occurring in Alzheimer's disease.

53. C   Abrupt onset is more likely in delirium.

54. B   Predictors of poor outcome in conduct disorder are: Low IQ, early onset (before 10 yrs of age), Family criminality and poor parenting. Poor educational achievements and low socio-economic status.

Bassarath L (2001) Can J Psychiatry.

55. C   Childhood schizophrenia is not included. PDD-NOS is another category included in DSM-IV.

Shaw JA (1999) J Am Acad Child Adol Psychiatry.

56. A   It is more common in females.

57. E   Few friends, absent or unavailable parents, stepfather and conflict with or between parents are primary markers for girl's sexual abuse.

The National Resource Centre on Child Sexual Abuse. (1994) The Incidence and Prevalence of Child Sexual Abuse, Hunstsville: NRCCSA.

58. D   More common in females after puberty, reverse is true for boys.

59. D   There is no evidence that early potty training prevents bedwetting. Risk factors include disturbed sleep; mother smokes at least 10 cigarettes a day at home and not being first born, neurological problems, UTI and constipation.

Touchette E, Petit D, Paquet J, et al (2005) Bed-wetting and its association with developmental milestones in early childhood. Arch Pediatr Adolesc. 159(12):1129-34.

60. C   ICD-10 code F93.0 is applicable.

The ICD-10 (1992) Classification of Mental and Behavioural Disorders. World Health Organization, Geneva.

61. A   There is no strong association with major mental illness.

62. D   It is usually associated with chronic constipation.

63. B   It is more common in males.

64. C   Pervasive anhedonia rarely occurs in children.

American Psychological Association (2003)- Oregon adolescent depression project.

65. D   The average age of onset is 60 years. Emotional and cognitive disorders are common in Parkinson's disease, but psychiatric disorders are not.

National Institute of Neurological Disorders and Stroke- 2007, USA.

66. B   DJ-1 is associated with Parkinson's disease.

67. B   Olfactory, tactile and kinaesthetic hallucinations are commonly seen in partial complex seizures. They are infrequently associated with psychosis, somotisation and schizophrenia.

68. E   There is strong association with previous depressive illness.

Companion to Psychiatric Studies -2004.

69. B   It is more common among Jewish people, elderly, lower social class and nursing & medical students.

70. A   Excessive energy is not associated. Other psychiatric features are irritability, memory impairment, negativism and social withdrawal. There is high prevalence of psychiatric symptoms in Addison's disease.

71. B   Epstein-Barr virus (EBV) is linked with CFS.

Afari N and Buchwald, D (2003) Chronic Fatigue Syndrome: A Review. Am J Psych 160:221-236.

72. D

73. A   Prevalence is 1 in 30 000 for male to female transsexuals and 1 in 100 000 for females to males transsexuals.

Sample D, et al (2005) Transsexualism -Oxford handbook of Psychiatry, Oxford.

74. C   Most patients will see dermatologist or plastic surgeon first than a psychiatrist.

75. E   There is however no clear evidence whether this is the cause or effect of delinquency.

76. D

77. D

HCR-20 manual version 2.

78. E

Department of Health (1990) The Care Programme Approach for people with a Mental Illness referred to the Specialist Psychiatrist Service.

79. D

Howells K et al; challenges in the treatment of dangerous and severe personality disorder: APT (2007).

80. E   In addition, mental state examination and certain other case specific investigations are also crucial to the assessment of dangerousness e.g. PCL-R, PPG etc.

Chiswick & Cope: Seminars in Practical Forensic Psychiatry 2001.

81. A   The commonest mode of death in prison is by suicide, which is almost always done by hanging. It is most common in remand prisoners. It is managed by segregating the prisoner.

Chiswick & Cope: Seminars in Practical Forensic Psychiatry 2001.

82. A   It is followed by the others in the order they have been listed in the question.

83. E   Prison population is generally from a disadvantaged background hence psychiatric conditions are fairly common. Psychiatric symptoms are common in the first two months of imprisonment and between third and a half may have ICD-10 classifiable disorder.

84. A

85. B

86. B

87. E

88. B

Bhaumik & Branford. The Frith prescribing guidelines for Adults with LD. Leicestershire Partnership NHS Trust. (2005).

89. B

Bhaumik & Branford. The Frith prescribing guidelines for Adults with LD. Leicestershire Partnership NHS Trust. (2005).

90. A This is caused by small deletion; Karyotype 16pter-p13.3 (cryptic terminal deletion); Clinical feature is LD.

91. E They usually take the form of "salaam attacks".

92. B It is an X-linked dominant condition.

93. A

94. A

95. C However if the first episode of depression is after 50 years of age then CT head should be done to exclude any organic cause.

96. E Other poor prognostic factors are enlarged ventricles and symptoms fulfilling more restrictive criteria.

97. E   There is no characteristic structural finding on neuroimaging in schizophrenia. However increased ventricle to brain ratio is the only consistent finding. The diagnosis nonetheless remains clinical at this stage.

Schmidt RA: Psychiatry Board Review, second edition (2006).

98. D

99. D   If during the process of discontinuation symptoms reoccur, revert to the effective dose and consider reduction after further stability of 6 months.

100. E   Others include MS, epilepsy, head injury, hyperthyroidism and hypothyroidism.

101. D   Other features of lithium toxicity are weakness, dizziness, nystagmus, nausea, vomiting and abdominal pain. In cases of severe toxicity blurred vision, circulatory shock, seizures and coma may occur.

102. E   It is an intense and prolonged grief reaction lasting over a year. Other symptoms include marked slowing of thoughts and movements.

Parkes CM. Bereavement: studies of grief in adult life. 2nd ed. (1986).

103. A

104. B   The volume reduction is 8% and is associated with short term memory loss.

105. A   A decrease in volume of caudate and abnormalities in prefrontal cortex have been noted.

Schmidt RA: Psychiatry Board Review, second edition (2006).

106. C   Neuroendocrine studies have revealed some overlaps between depression and OCD.

107. D Mortality rate in anorexia nervosa is 10 to 15%.

Semple et al: Oxford Handbook of Psychiatry (2005).

108. A Self help manuals and Psychoeducation are useful as first step. IPT may be as effective as CBT in long term but takes longer to show response.

109. D

110. C Bupropion is also reported to increase sex drive.

111. C Long term admission is of little benefit in personality disorder. They usually benefit from admissions for axis I disorder or in crisis, which are usually brief.

Davison SE. Principles of managing patients with personality disorder. APT (2002).

112. E Cluster A patients generally worsen, Cluster B improve and Cluster C stay the same with age. 50% of schizotypal personality disorder patients develop schizophrenia over time.

Tyrer & Seivewright, Outcome of personality disorder. In personality disorders: diagnosis, management and cause. Ed. Tyrer P. Oxford: Butterworth Heinemann (2000).

113. C It should be treated with psychological support and antidepressants.

Whitehead et al. Antidepressants for the treatment of depression in people with schizophrenia: a systematic review. Psycho Med (2003).

114. A Its other main uses are service evaluation, promoting effective service development and keeping an overview of patient's unmet needs from both his perspective and service perspective.

Davenport S. Ensuring the community care: assessment and evaluation of social care needs in long-term mental illness. APT (2006).

115. A

Adshead & Ferris, Treatment of victims of trauma: APT (2007).

116. A Treatment should be continued for at least 5 years or indefinitely if the episodes have been very severe. Risk of relapse is 70 90 % if medication is stopped before 5 years.

117. A

118. C Its prognosis is better than that for schizophrenia but significantly worse than that for mood disorders. The good/poor prognostic factors are however the same as that for schizophrenia.

119. A Other good prognostic factors are few thoughts of suicide, good treatment response and compliance.

120. B Monotherapy with lamotrigine is supported by evidence to be used in refractory bipolar depression. Other alternative is an addition of triiodothyronine in absence hypothyroidism. Inositol may also be used as an adjunctive therapy.

Calabrese JR et al. Latest maintenance data on lamotrigine in bipolar disorder: Eur Neuropsychopharmacol (2003).
Bauer M et al. Supraphysiological doses of L-thyroxine in the maintenance treatment of prophylaxis-resistant affective disorders. Neuropsychopharmacol (2002).

121. E

122. B

123. B Other factors include late age of onset, excessive weight loss, anxiety while eating with others and history of difficult childhood. With treatment anorexia will recover fully in a third, partial remission in a third and will be resistant with chronic problems in a third of cases.

124. B   Severe personality disorder and low self-esteem can impede the otherwise good prognosis of bulimia nervosa.

125. A   It is treated with stimulants and regular naps in the day. Cataplexy which is one of its clinical features may be treated with SSRIs or tricyclic antidepressants. Abrupt withdrawal of medication may lead to status cataplectcus.

Ohayon MM et al, Prevelance of narcolepsy symptomatology and diagnosis in the European general population: Neurology (2002).

126. E   There is no clear evidence that medication has any direct effect on personality disorder itself, any benefit seen by pharmacological therapy is probably due to its effect on any comorbid axis I disorder.

Tyrer P. Drug treatment of personality disorder. In personality disorders: diagnosis, management and cause. Ed. Tyrer P. Oxford: Butterworth Heinemann (2000).

127. B   Abnormal Involuntary Movement Scale (AIMS) should ideally be used every six months to examine and monitor a patient on long term antipsychotic treatment for development of extrapyramidal side effects.

Munetz & Benjamin. How to examine patients using the Abnormal Involuntary Movement Scale. Hospital and Community Psychiatry (1988).

128. A   There is also some evidence for CBT, compliance therapy and depot medication in reducing relapse rate. In case of the latter patients non attendance for the injection can be an early sign of relapse hence prompting early intervention.
Nadeem et al. Schizophrenia. Clinical Evidence (2003).

129. B   Spinal injuries cause erectile dysfunction instead of loss of libido. Management of reduced libido includes treating the primary cause, addressing relationship issues and if required, behavioural therapy and sensate focus techniques may also be used.

Masters & Johnson. Human sexual response. New York: Bantam Books.

130. E Trichotillomania is an obsession with pulling ones hair, which relieves stress. It is usually exacerbated by stress but at times even relaxation can trigger it. SSRIs, lithium, clomipramine, pimozide and risperidone have some evidence in its treatment.

Walsh & McDougle. Trichotillomania: presentation, etiology, diagnosis and therapy. Am J Clin Dermatol. (2001).

131-133. A, C and F.

134-136. C, E and G

137-139. B, F and H

140-142. A, E and F

143-145. A, D and G

146. E

147. H

148. F

149. G

150-151. A, C

152-153. B, D

154-155. E, H

156. E

157. F

158. G

159. B

160. A

161. G

162. C

163. B

164-165. C, H

166-167. B, E

168-169. A, D

170-171. F, J

172-173. G, I

174. E

175. H

176. C

177. D

178. A

179. E

180. E

181. I

182. B

183. H

184-185. E, G

186-187. D, F

188-189. B, H

190. A

191. B

192. D

193. A

194. C

195. B

196. C

197. A

198. A

199. D

200. B

References and Further Reading

1. Shorter Oxford Textbook of Psychiatry Michael G, 2006. Oxford university press.

2. Kaplan & Sadock's Comprehensive Textbook of Psychiatry 7th edition 2000, Lippincott Williams & Wilkins. USA.

3. Oxford Handbook of Psychiatry 2005, Semple, D. OUP Oxford.

4. Chiswisk & Cope: Seminars in Practical Forensic Psychiatry 2001.

5. Critical Appraisal for Psychiatrists, S Lawrie. 2000. Churchill Livingstone.

6. Bhaumik & Branford: The Frith Prescribing Guidelines for Adults with LD. 2005.

7. The Doctor's guide to Critical Appraisal, 2006. N Gosall. Pas Test.

8. Sackett DL, et al 2000 Evidence Based Medicine, 2nd edition. Churchill-Livingstone, London).

9. Freedman D 2005, statistical models: Theory and practice. Cambridge University Press.

10. Wasserman L 2007, All of Non Parametric statistics, Springer.

11.   Hollis S and Campbell F, 1991 BMJ, 319:670-74.

12.   Nikulin MS and Greenwood PE,1996   A Guide to Chi Squared testing New York: Wiley Inter science.

13.   Statistics Glossary v1.1, Valerie J. Easton and John H. McColl.

14.   Richard A Berk, Regression Analysis: A Constructive Critique, sage Publication. 2004.

15.   Dickerson K, JAMA 1990; 263(10):1385-9.

16.   Michel Ibrahim et al Dec 1999, Eric notebook.

17.   Gardner & Altman 1989.

18.   Jerald F. Lawless. Statistical Models and Methods for Lifetime Data, 2nd edition. John Wiley and Sons, Hoboken. 2003.

19.   Drummond, Stoddart and Torrance 1987.

20.   Christine Brown and Keith Llyod, APT 2001, 7:350-356.

21.   Edwards G and Gross MM 1976, Alcohol dependence: provisional description of a clinical syndrome. BMJ 1, 1058-61.

22.   Towards a comprehensive model of change, Changing for Good, JO Prochaska, J Norcross & DiClimente Sep 1995, First Avon books.

23.   Wright T, Myrick H, Henderson S, Peters H, Malcolm R. Risk factors for delirium tremens: a retrospective chart review. Am J Addict. May-Jun 2006;15(3):213-9.

24.   BMJ 2003, 183:304-313.

25.   Littleton 2007, Journal of addiction medicine 1(3) 115-125.

26.   Gau S.S.F et al 2004 BJP 185: 422-428.

27.   Arseneault et al 2004.

28.   Robert L Palmer, APT 2002, vol 8, pp.10-16.

29.   Ryle 1990 and 1995.

30.   Clinician's quick guide to interpersonal psychotherapy.
       New York: Oxford University Press.

31.   Weissman, M. M, Markowitz, J. C., & Klerman, G. L. (2007).

32.   Primary Care Companion J Clin Psychiatry 2000;2:1315.

33.   Pietro, Calif Med. 1967 September; 107(3): 263269).

34.   Scogin &McElreath 1994.

35.   Freud, A. (1937). The Ego and the Mechanisms of Defence.
       London: Hogarth Press and Institute of Psycho-Analysis.

36.   Cramer, P. (1991). The Development of Defence
       Mechanisms: Theory, Research, and Assessment. New
       York, Springer-Verlag.

37.   Significant aspects of Client centred therapy, Carl Rogers. 1946.

38.   Ref: Alan M & Susie V M. APT 2008, 14: 42-49.

39.   Jeremy Holmes, APT 1994, vol 1, p. 9-15.

40.   Applegate B et al. 1997 J Am Acad Child Adol Psychiatry.

41.   Schneider JH and Glaze DG (2002).

42. Rapoport JL, Inoff-Germain G (2000) J Child Psychol Psychiat.

43. Scahill L, Williams S, Schwab-Stone M, Applegate J, Leckman JF.(2006) Disruptive behavior problems in a community sample of children with tic disorders. Adv Neurol. ;99:184-90.

44. Cawson, P., Wattam, C., Brooker, S., and Kelly, G. (2000) Child maltreatment in the United Kingdom: a study of the prevalence of child abuse and neglect. London: NSPCC.

45. Rutter M (2005)Incidence of autism spectrum disorders: changes over time and their meaning. Acta Paediatr 94 (1): 215.

46. Fetal Alcohol Syndrome(2004) : Guidelines for Referral and Diagnosis.CDC.

47. Adams JA, (2004) Medical evaluation of suspected child sexual abuse. J Pediatr Adolesc Gynecol.17(3): 191-7.

48. Shepherd, J.P.; Sutherland, I.; Newcombe, R.G. (2006)Relations between alcohol, violence and victimization in adolescence. Journal of Adolescence, 29(4): 539-553.

49. Carr, A. (ed.) (2000) What Works with Children and Adolescents?- A Critical Review of Psychological Interventions with Children, Adolescents and their Families. London: Brunner-Routledge.

50. The Royal College of Psychiatrists-Factsheet 9: Children Who Do Not Go To School.

51. Butler RJ, Golding J, Northstone K (2005) Nocturnal enuresis at 7.5 years old: prevalence and analysis of clinical signs. BJU Int.(3):404-10.

52.   Goldner EM, Hsu L, Waraich P, Somers JM (2002) Prevalence and incidence studies of schizophrenic disorders: a systematic review of the literature. Canadian Journal of Psychiatry, 47(9), 83343.

53.   Astley, S.J. (2004). Diagnostic Guide for Fetal Alcohol Spectrum Disorders: The 4-Digit Diagnostic Code. Seattle: University of Washington.

54.   Denckla MB (2006) Attention deficit hyperactivity disorder: the childhood co-morbidity that most influences the disability burden in Tourette syndrome. Adv Neurol. 99:1721.

55.   ICD-10 (1992) the International Statistical Classification of Diseases and Related Health Problems, WHO.

56.   Schreier H (2002) Munchausen by proxy defined. Pediatrics.110 :985 988.

57.   Boeing L, Murray V, Pelosi A, McCabe R, Blackwood D and Wrate R (2007) Adolescent-onset psychosis: prevalence, needs and service provision. British Journal of Psychiatry, 198, 18-26.

58.   Fellick et al (2001) Neurological soft signs in mainstream pupils Arch Dis Child. 85: 371-374.

59.   Mayoclinic.com (2007)- Childhood schizophrenia.

60.   MedicineNet.com (2003)- Methylphenidate.

61.   Royal College of Psychiatrists (2004) Factsheet 14: Divorce or seperation of parents - the impact on children and adolescents.

62.   George C Patton et al.(2002)Cannabis use and mental health in young people: cohort study. BMJ, 325:1195-1198.

63.   Kovacs M, et als (1997) Psychiatric disorders in youths with IDDM: rates and risk factors. Diabetes care. 20(1): 36-44.

64.   Neary D et als. (1998) Frontotemporal lobar degeneration: a consensus on clinical diagnostic criteria." 'Neurology' 51(6):1546-

65.   Waldemar G, Dubois B, Emre M, et al (2007). "Recommendations for the diagnosis and management of Alzheimer's disease and other disorders associated with dementia: EFNS guideline". Eur. J. Neurol. 14 (1): e126.

66.   Bird, T. D. "Memory loss and dementia." In Harrison's Principles of Internal.

67.   Medicine, 15th edition, A. S. Franci, E. Daunwald, and K. J. Isrelbacher, eds.

68.   NewYork: McGraw Hill, 2001.

69.   Tang W, Chan S, Chiu H et als (2004). Impact of applying NINDS-AIREN.

70.   criteria of probable vascular dementia to clinical and radiological characteristics of a stroke cohort with dementia". Cerebrovasc. Dis. 18 (2): 98-103.

71.   Hachinski VC, Iliff LD, Zilhka E et als. (1975)Cerebral blood flow in.

72.   dementia.Arch Neurol;32:632-7.

73.   Lyketsos C, Colenda C, Beck C, et als (2006). Position statement of the American Association for Geriatric Psychiatry (AAGP) regarding principles of care for patients with dementia resulting from Alzheimer disease. Am J Geriatr Psychiatry 14 (7): 561-72.

74.   J. Xie, C. Brayne, F. E Matthews, and the Medical Research Council Cognitive Function (2008). Survival times in people with dementia: analysis from population based cohort study with 14 year follow-up. BMJ, January 10, 2008 bmj.39433.616678.25v1.

75.   Cole G M and Dendukuri N (2003) Risk Factors for Depression Among Elderly Community Subjects: A Systematic Review and Meta-Analysis. Am J Psychiatry 160:1147-1156.

76.   Conrad C, Andreadis A, Trojanowski JQ, et als (1997) Genetic Evidence For the Involvement Of Tau In Progressive Supranuclear Palsy. Annals of Neurology 41: 277-281.

77.   Jesse Dukeminier & Stanley M. Johanson (2005) Wills, Trusts & Estates, Sixth Edition, Aspen Publishers.

78.   Bateman GA, Levi CR, Schofield P, et al (2005) the pathophysiology of the aqueduct stroke volume in normal pressure hydrocephalus: can co-morbidity with other forms of dementia be excluded? Neuroradiology, 47(10): 741-8.

79.   Dombrovski, Alexandre Y1; Szanto, Katalin; Reynolds III, Charles F (2005) Epidemiology and risk factors for suicide in the elderly: 10-year update.Aging Health, Volume 1, Number 1:135-145.

80.   Dalfen AK, Anthony F. Head injury (2000) dissociation and the Ganser syndrome. Brain Inj ;14(12):1101-5.

81.   Manela, M., Katona, C. & Livingston, G. (1996) How common are the anxiety.

82.   Disorders in old age? International Journal of Geriatric Psychiatry, 6, 6570.

83.   Levinoff JE (2007)Vascular Dementia and Alzheimer's
       Disease: Diagnosis and Risk Factors. Geriatrics
       Aging;10(1):36-41.

84.   Nagaratnam N, Bou-Haidar P, Leung H (2003)Confused
       and disturbed behaviour in the elderly following silent
       frontal lobe infarction.. Am J Alzheimers Dis Other
       Demen:18 (6):333-9.

85.   Wright T, Myrick H, Henderson S, Peters H, Malcolm R
       (2006) Risk factors for delirium tremens: a retrospective
       chart review. Am J Addict;15 (3):213-9.

86.   Uchihara, T; Ikeda K, Tsuchiya K (2003) Pick body disease
       and Pick syndrome.". Neuropathology 23 (4): 318-326.

87.   Brown, R. G. & Marsen, C. D. (1988) Sub-cortical dementia:
       the neuropsychological evidence. Neuroscience, 25, 363-387.

88.   Takeda K; ;Rinsho Shinkeigaku.(2004),44(11):834-6.

89.   Östling, Svante (2005) Psychotic symptoms in the elderly.
       Current Psychosis & Therapeutics Reports 3:1.

90.   Morris MC, Evans DA, Schneider JA, et als.(2006). Dietary
       folate and vitamins B-12 and B-6 not associated with
       incident Alzheimer's disease. J. Alzheimers Dis. 9 (4): 435-43.

91.   Adams et al., Dysmnesic Syndrome, Alcohol-Induced.
       Principles of Neurology, 6th ed, p1139.

92.   Goscinski I, Kwiatkowski S, Polak J, et al.(1997) The
       Kluver-Bucy syndrome. J Neurosurg Sci;41(3):269-72.

93.   E. Gomez-Tortosa, A. et als.(1998) Severity of Cognitive
       Impairment in Juvenile and Late-Onset Huntington
       DiseaseArch Neurol: 55(6): 835 843.

94.   Stone J, Carson A, Sharpe M., 2005, Functional symptoms in neurology: Assessment, Journal of Neurology, Neurosurgery and Psychiatry (Neurology in Practice); 76 (Suppl 1): 2-12.

96.   National Institute of Neurological Disorders and Stroke,- 2008, USA.

97.   Petronis A (1999) Alzheimer's disease and Down syndrome: From Meiosis to Dementia. Experimental Neurology, Volume 158, Number 2, pp. 403-413.

98.   Curyto K J et als (2001) Survival of Hospitalized Elderly Patients With Delirium: A Prospective Study. American Journal of Geriatric Psychiatry 9; 141-147.

99.   Sang Kun Lee, et als (2005) Occipital Lobe Epilepsy: Clinical Characteristics, Surgical Outcome, and Role of Diagnostic Modalities. Epilepsia, Volume 46, Issue 5, Page 688-695.

100.   Medline Plus-(2006) Somatization disorder.

104.   Cryer P, Slone R, Whyte M (1996)Depression and hypercalcemia. Clinicopathologic Conference. Am J Med.101(1):111-7.

105.   Ainiala H, Loukkola J, Peltola J, et al(2001) The prevalence of neuropsychiatric syndromes in systemic lupus erythematosus. Neurology. 57(3):496-500.

108.   Andreoli T, et al. (1993) Cecil Essentials of Medicine. 3rd ed. Philadelphia, Pa.

110.   Fukao A, Takamatsu J, Murakami Y(2003) The relationship of psychological factors to the prognosis of hyperthyroidism in antithyroid drug-treated patients with Graves" disease. Clin Endocrinol (Oxf).58(5):550-5.

111.   Katharine A. Phillips (2007) Suicidality in Body
        Dysmorphic Disorder Primary Psychiatry.14 (12):58-66.

112.   Day, E., Bentham, P., Callagham, R. et al. (2004) Thiamine
        for the WernickeKorsakoff Syndrome in people at risk
        from alcohol abuse (Cochrane Review). In The Cochrane
        Library, issue 2. John Wiley & Sons Ltd, Chichester, UK.

113.   Vinken PJ, et als . Handbook of clinical neurology. Vol-55,
        Elsevier Science Publishers, Amsterdam.

114.   Waldrop-Valverde (2005) Influence of depression and
        HIV serostatus on the neuropsychological performance of
        injecting drug users. Psych Clin Neurosci:59(4) 372-8.

119.   125-American association on mental Retardation (1992).

120.   Bregman JD and Volkmer FR. Journal of Am Acad of Child
        and Adol. (1998).

122.   Skuse & Mandy. Measuring autistic traits: heritability,
        reliability and validity of the Social and Communication
        Disorders Checklist. BJP (2005).

123.   Welsh Health Survey. Welsh Office, Cardiff (1995).

124.   Mariani et al. Epilepsy in institutionalized patients with
        encephalopathy: Clinical aspects and nosological
        considerations. Am. J. Ment. Retardation (1993).

125.   Menéndez M. Review article. Down syndrome,
        Alzheimer's disease and seizures. Brain and Development
        (2005).

127.   Lennox H Huang. Williams Syndrome. eMedicine
        Specialties (2006).

128.   Cassidy SB. Prader-Willi syndrome Journal of Med Genet

(1997).

129. Crawford et al. FMR1 and the Fragile X syndrome: Human genome epidemiology review. Genet Med (2001).

130. Stratton et al. Foetal Alcohol Syndrome: Diagnosis, Epidemiology, Prevention, and Treatment. Institute of Medicine (IOM), Washington, DC: National Academy Press (1996).

131. Roizen & Patterson. Down's syndrome. Lancet. (2003).

132. Girirajan et al. Genotype-phenotype correlation in Smith-Magenis syndrome: evidence that multiple genes in 17p11.2 contribute to the clinical spectrum. Genet Med (2006).

133. Bhaumik & Branford. The Frith prescribing guidelines for Adults with LD. Leicestershire Partnership NHS Trust. (2005).

134. The Maudsley prescribing guidelines (2008).

135. Chiswick & Cope: Seminars in Practical Forensic Psychiatry (2001).

137. HCR-20 manual version 2.

138. Lipsedge, M.(1995) Psychiatry: reducing risk in clinical practice. In Clinical Risk Management (ed. C. Vincent).

139. Department of Health (1990) The Care Programme Approach for people with a Mental Illness referred to the Specialist Psychiatrist Service.

140. National Confidential Inquiry into Suicide & Homicide by People with Mental Illness: Safer Services 1999.

141.   Kennedy H.G (2002) APT: Therapeutic uses of security: Mapping Forensic Mental Health Services by Stratifying Risk.

142.   Royal College of Psychiatrists (1995) Strategies for the Management of Disturbed and Violent Patients in Psychiatric Units (Council Report CR41).

143.   Riordan S. et al (2004) The imposition of restricted hospital orders: Potential effects of ethnic origin. International Journal of Law and Psychiatry.

144.   Meyer JM. Individual changes in clozapine levels after smoking cessation: results and a predictive model. J Clin Psychopharmacol. 2001.

145.   Flanagan & Spencer: (1999) Therapeutic monitoring of clozapine and norclozapine. CPMS Newsletter.

146.   Flanagan & Spencer: A Practical Approach to the Therapeutic Monitoring of Clozapine.

147.   Department of Health. Reforming The Mental Health Act.2000.

149.   Home Office (1992) Gender and The Criminal Justice System. London: HMSO.

150.   Gibson, E. (1975) Homicide in England & Wales 1967- 71. Home Office Research Study no 31. London. HMSO.

151.   Meadow, R. (1989) Munchausen Syndrome by Proxy: BMJ.

152.   Mullen, P; Schizophrenia and violence: from correlations to preventive strategies. APT 2006.

153.   Howells K et al; challenges in the treatment of dangerous and severe personality disorder: APT(2007).

154. Monahan J (1984) The prediction of violent behaviour: towards a second generation of theory and policy. AJP.

155. GMC; Confidentiality: protecting and providing information (2004).

156. Schmidt RA: Psychiatry Board Review, second edition (2006).

157. Ferrier IN: Water intoxication in patients with psychiatric illness. BMJ (1985).

158. Levenson JL. Neuroleptic Malignant Syndrome. AJP (1985).

159. NICE Guidelines on the use of Electroconvulsive therapy (May 2003).

160. Mukherjee S et al. Electroconvulsive therapy of acute manic episodes: a review of 50 years experience. AJP (1994).

161. American Psychiatric Association. Practice guideline for the treatment of patients with bipolar disorder. AJP (1994).

162. Ballenger JC et al. Panic attack and agoraphobia. Treatments of psychiatric disorders, 2nd ed. Vol 2. American Psychiatric Pess, Washington DC (1997).

163. Wolpe J. The practice of behaviour therapy. 2nd ed. Pergamon. New York (1973).

164. McElroy SL et al. Kleptomania: a report of 20 cases. AJP (1991).

165. Schenck & Mahowald. REM sleep behaviour disorder: clinical, developmental and neuroscience perspectives 16 years after its formal identification in SLEEP. Sleep (2002).

166.   Davison SE. Principles of managing patients with personality disorder. APT (2002).

167.   Adshead G. Psychiatric staff as attachment figures. Understanding management problems in psychiatric services in the light of attachment theory. BJP (1998).

168.   Davison & Tyrer. Psychosocial treatment in personality disorder. In personality disorders: diagnosis, management and cause. Ed. Tyrer P. Oxford: Butterworth Heinemann (2000).

169.   Ziegenbein et al. Augmentation of clozapine with amisulpride in patients with treatment resistant schizophrenia. An open clinical study. GJP (2006).

170.   Palmer B. Come the revolution. Revisiting: the management of anorexia nervosa. APT (2006).

171.   Davenport S. Ensuring the community cares: assessment and evaluation of social care needs in long term mental illness. APT (2006).

172.   Mitchell & Selmes. Why don't patients take their medicine? Reasons and solutions in psychiatry. APT (2007).

173.   Rinaldi & Perkins. Vocational rehabilitation. Psychiatry (2004).

174.   Crowther et al. Helping people with severe mental illness to obtain work: systematic review. BMJ (2001).

175.   Hoff et al. Neuropsychology in schizophrenia: an update. Schizophrenia. Current Opinion in Psychiatry. (2003).

176.   Johnstone, E C, Eds: Companion to Psychiatric Studies. 7th Edition (2004).

177.   Michael A, Ed (2004)-Get Through MRCPsych Parts 1 &2:1001 EMIQs.

178.   Patel AG (2006)-The complete MRCPsych Part-2.

179.   NICE Guidelines for Schizophrenia (2002).

180.   There are several courses, course materials and websites that we have found helpful in the past preparing for exams, gaining knowledge and even now that knowledge has been very useful in compiling this book. Some worth mentioning are super-ego café, Manchester course, Birmingham course and trickcyclists.co.uk.

181.   www.rcpsych.ac.uk.

182.   www.acat.me.uk.

183.   www.dvla.gov.uk.

184.   Www.cebm.net.